GREEN MOUNTAIN

WOOD PELLET GRILL

COOKBOOK

1000-DAY EASY BBQ RECIPE FOR YOUR GREEN MOUNTAIN WOOD PELLET GRILL

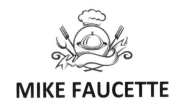

MIKE FAUCETTE

CONTENTS

INTRODUCTION

What IS Green Mountain Wood Pellet Grill?

Wood Pellet grills utilize ignited wood pellets and a system of fans to heat food to a specific temperature, quite like an outdoor convection oven. Pellet grills can be used to smoke, grill, bake and even braise food. Nearly anything you make in a standard oven can be made on a pellet grill.

How does Green Mountain Wood Pellet Grill work?

The heat is generated from wood pellets that are placed in a chamber called a "pellet hopper." Those pellets move through an auger to a fire pot, which heats the entire cooking chamber of the grill. Through a fan system, heat and smoke are dispensed throughout the grill, providing a naturally rich and woody flavor from the pellets. Though pellet grills certainly share some characteristics of your traditional grills, there are a couple of major differences that set pellet grills apart: most notably, the combination of deep flavor, versatility and efficiency.

Why People Choose the Green Mountain Wood Pellet Grill?

1.Green Mountain WOOD PELLET GRILL IS EASY TO USE

One of the greatest features of a pellet grill is the fact they're easy to use. Simply fill the hopper with food-grade wood pellets, empty the ash pail, and select your desired temperature and smoke level. The pellet grill takes over from there as an electric auger feeds the burn pot with wood pellets from the hopper.

Once you set the temperature, the pellet grill maintains it and feeds wood pellets as needed. Pellet grills are highly precise with temperature control from their lowest to highest settings (180-500 degrees on many grills).

For even more accurate control, grill blankets are available to help pellet grills hold in more heat and smoke. They maintain even more consistent temperatures throughout the entire year, but they're especially useful in the winter months when outside temperatures drop.

Pellet grills are also easy to clean when you're finished cooking. Whether it's a quick clean-up or a deeper clean, no effort takes longer than 15 minutes to maintain your grill.

2. SET IT & FORGET IT

With pellet grills, you can set it and walk away. Since the grill does all the work, you get a wood-fired taste without having to constantly feed logs or wood chunks. Overall, pellet grills do not require as much time or attention, and there's no need to constantly check the grill temperature or level of smoke.

Newer models even monitor temperature levels from the palm of your hand. Traeger and Camp Chef now both feature, easy-to-use, WiFi controlling technology. Change the temperature, adjust smoke levels, and receive notifications from your phone.

3. VERSATILITY TO COOK ANYTHING

Naturally, a pellet grill is great for smoking and grilling, but it's also the centerpiece for much more. All of your favorite dishes that are usually cooked inside can now be done outdoors. Think of it as a kitchen in your backyard where you can perfectly cook anything with confidence.

➤ **BBQ**

Traditional smokers have set the BBQ bar for a long time and are debated to provide a better smoke. On the opposite side of that argument are pellet grills. Pellet grills are now recognized for their quality and are even sanctioned in contests sponsored by the Kansas City Barbeque Society (KCBS), winning many bbq competitions in recent years.

The combination of smoke quality and convenience with pellet grills is unbeatable. Taste all of your barbecue favorites from the comfort of your own backyard. Pick your favorite wood pellet flavors, set the grill on low and go. You'll love the beautiful smoke ring, tenderness, and delicious flavor you get from home cooked ribs, pulled pork, beef brisket, chicken quarters and wings. Fresh salmon, trout, and even sides such as mac and cheese are wonderfully smoky and tasty.

➤ **BAKE**

Anything cooked in an oven can be done in a pellet grill. Pellet grills primarily work as a convection oven. Indirect heat and smoke are produced from the burn pot and blown around the pellet grill for a perfect, evenly cooked finish. Bake breads, cakes, pies, breakfast casseroles, and delicious, wood-fired pizzas. Plus, when you bake your favorites outside in the summer months, you avoid heating up your house and kitchen.

➢ GRILL

For many of our common grilling favorites–such as summer burgers and hot dogs–there's a time when we need to turn up the heat. Pork chops and your favorite cuts of steak or chicken are fabulous when cooked over a wood fire. Don't forget your vegetables too!

Pellet grills used to only have an indirect heat option, but that has changed in recent years. To improve the grilling feature, many manufacturers now offer models with perforated drip trays, direct heat over the burn pot, and/or temperatures up to 500°. This allows your burgers and steaks to sizzle and get those beautiful grill marks and a good crust on the outside, while still preserving a medium to rare center.

4. GREAT WOOD-FIRED FLAVORS

While there are many grilling options out there, nothing produces better tasting food than a pellet grill. Fuel flavors your food and with wood-fired flavors are superior to gas and charcoal alternatives. All of your favorite dishes are simply better on a pellet grill.

With pellet grills, you also have flavor options when choosing wood pellets for your grill. Each pellet flavor, or type of wood, has a unique taste that naturally complements and enhances your favorite foods. Specific hardwood blends are also available. Experiment with different food-grade wood pellet options and find the flavors you and your family enjoy the most.

How to Use the Green Mountain Wood Pellet Grill?

For wood pellet newcomers, pellet grills and smokers are an excellent way to get into barbecue. Learn how to get the best out of your wood cooker with our step-by-step guide to using a pellet smoker grill.

1. Season your pellet smoker.

Before we do anything, we need to season the smoker. This is a crucial step for any type of new smoker, and helps protect it from the negative effects of long term continuous use. The basic premise is to apply cooking oil to the grates and inside of the chamber and then take the smoker on a 'dry run' without food. This will cook the oil onto the inside surfaces of the smoker, forming a protective layer across it.

After you have seasoned it, leave the smoker to cool and rest for at least 24 hours before using properly.

2. Preheat your smoker.

A big pain with charcoal grills is heating them up. Lighting them and keeping them at a good temperature can be tricky. Not so with a pellet grill. They work much in the same way as an oven.

With your grill plugged in to an electric outlet or socket, switch it on and select your target temperature. If you're going for barbecue smoking, choose 225°F (107°C).

Most smokers will take about 10 minutes to preheat and come to temperature.

You should hear a dull roar come from the smoker as it heats up. This is the motorized auger and firebox springing into action, and is a good sign that your smoker is working and warming up.

Pro tip: While pellet smokers do have a temperature gauge on their control display, it's not unusual for these to be inaccurate by up to about 20°F either way. Get a dual probe smoker thermometer. These allow you to simultaneously measure cooking and internal meat temperatures. The best models are more accurate than the majority of built-in gauges.

3. Add your meat.

With your pellet smoker now running at target temperature, carefully place your meat on the smoker grates. For the best results, place the food in the middle of the grate. This will ensure that the meat is far away enough from the heat to not dry out, but close enough to be cooked at temperature.

4. Pay attention to fat content.

A mistake that a lot of BBQ newcomers make is with the meat itself. Meat that is too lean can dry out quickly, whereas meat with too much fat content can get in the way of the smoke working its way into the flesh of the meat.

If you choose to smoke a cut like brisket, then be sure that you trim the layer of fat on it to about ½ inch thick before putting it on the smoker.

How to Clean and Care for Your Green Mountain Wood Pellet Grill?

➢ **BETWEEN EACH COOK**

For quick cleanup between cookouts, you don't need to do anything too dramatic. In fact, our patented Ash Cleanout system makes it as simple as pulling a knob. Before you fire up the grill each time, just empty the ash into the cup, and you're good to go. It's almost too easy.

Don't forget about the internal temperature probe. You'll want to clean it between each cook. It's located on the right side of the cooking chamber and is about the size of a pencil. Our goal is to keep it looking silver. To do this mixt a vinegar/water solution and use a scouring pad. Often times if your temperature does not read accurately it's because too much smoke has been build up.

Besides emptying the burn cup, you may want to spot clean between cook sessions as well. This can be as simple as wiping away grease spots or food residue on the lid or side shelf. You should also scrape down the grill grates with a wire grill brush or spatula before you start cooking to avoid a burnt taste on your food.

If you take these small steps toward keeping your pellet grill clean, any deeper cleaning you do will be much easier.

➢ **EXTERIOR**

Safety first! Make sure your grill is totally cool, then unplug it from its power source.

Empty the pellet hopper to prevent your pellets from getting wet or coming into contact with cleaning substances.

Spray stainless steel cleaner on the painted or stainless steel surfaces of your grill. Avoid spraying any plastic components. (You can also use hot, soapy water-it just may not work as quickly!)

Let the cleaner sit for about 30 seconds to give it a chance to break down grease and smoke stains.

Wipe off the cleaner with a clean paper towel or rag. Wipe with the grain if you're cleaning stainless steel or in circles, if you're cleaning a painted surface.

Repeat the process once more to clean off any remaining grease or smoke. With a rag, rinse thoroughly if you used soapy water.

Allow to dry for at least 24 hours before cooking, and double-check that the hopper has no water in it before reloading pellets.

➤ INTERIOR

Pull the Ash Cleanout knob and empty the ash from the burn cup.

Open the lid and remove the cooking grate, any extra racks, drip tray, and heat diffuser plate from inside the grill. Pay attention to how these pieces are installed (or even take a picture) so you'll have an easier time reassembling your grill.

Use a wet/dry vacuum with a hose attachment to remove loose ash and debris.

Look for places inside your grill where grease has built up. Use something with a flat edge (a paint stick, pan scraper, etc.) to dislodge and remove it.

Use hot, soapy water and a rag you aren't attached to wash the interior of your grill, as well as each piece you pulled out.

Repeat the process until most of the grease buildup is gone.

With a rag, rinse thoroughly if you used soapy water and allow everything to dry.

Cover the heat diffuser plate and drip tray with aluminum foil for easier cleaning next time (you can simply throw away and replace the foil rather than scrubbing off the grease).

Allow to dry for at least 24 hours before cooking, and double-check that the hopper has no water in it before reloading pellets.

BAKING RECIPES

Smoked Lemon Tea

Servings: 6 - 8

Cooking Time: 60 Minutes

Ingredients:
- 8 Black Tea Bags
- 4 Cups Boiling Water
- 2 Cups Ice
- 8 Lemons
- 2 Cups Sugar
- 2 Cups Water

Directions:

1. Place the tea bags in a heat-safe pitcher. Bring 4 Cups of water to a boil and pour over tea bags. Let steep for 5-10 minutes. Remove tea bags and set pitcher aside to cool.

2. Turn on your grill and set to smoke mode. Combine 2 cups of sugar and 2 cups water in a small aluminum pan. Smoke for about 45 minutes, stirring occasionally, or until the mixture reduces to a thick, simple syrup. Remove from the grill and let it cool.

3. Supply your smoker with wood pellets and follow the start-up procedure. Preheat the grill, with the lid closed, to 450° F. If using a charcoal or gas grill, set heat to high.

4. Cut the lemons in half and sear over the flame broiler until charred, about 7 minutes. Remove from grill and set aside to cool.

5. Juice the lemons into a medium bowl. Pour lemon juice through a metal strainer into the tea pitcher to remove seeds and pulp.

6. Pour the cooled simple syrup into pitcher and stir until fully incorporated with tea and lemons. Add 2 cups of ice and refrigerate until serving.

Sweet And Spicy Baked Pork Beans

Servings: 20

Cooking Time: 120 Minutes

Ingredients:

- ➢ 1 - 21 Oz Apple Pie Filling, Can
- ➢ 1 Gallon Baked Beans
- ➢ 1 Tbs Chilli, Powder
- ➢ 1 Green Bell Pepper, Diced
- ➢ 1 10 Oz Drained Jalapeno, Can Diced
- ➢ 1 Cup Maple Syrup
- ➢ 1 Onion, Diced
- ➢ 1 Lb Pork, Pulled

Directions:

1. Supply your smoker with wood pellets and follow the start-up procedure. Preheat the grill, with the lid closed, to 350° F.
2. Place all ingredients in mixing bowl and mix well.
3. Pour bean mixture into foil pans.
4. Bake in grill till bubbling throughout – about 2 hours.
5. Rest at least 15 minutes before serving.

Cherry Ice Cream Cobbler

Servings: 8

Cooking Time: 45 Minutes

Ingredients:

- ➢ 1 Tsp Baking Powder
- ➢ 3 Tbsp Butter, Melted
- ➢ 1 Cup Flour
- ➢ Ice Cream, Prepared
- ➢ 1/4 Tsp Salt
- ➢ 3/4 Cup Sugar
- ➢ 1/2 Cup Milk

Directions:

1. Supply your smoker with wood pellets and follow the start-up procedure. Preheat the grill, with the lid closed, to 350° F.

2. In a bowl, combine flour, sugar, baking powder, salt and mix to incorporate. Stir in butter and milk and mix until combined. In a cast iron pan, dump in cherry pie filling and pile on the prepared topping to cover.

3. Place in your Grill and bake for about 45 minutes, or until the topping is golden brown.

4. Let cool for a couple minutes and serve with ice cream.

Mint Butter Chocolate Chip Cookies

Servings: 24

Cooking Time: 12 Minutes

Ingredients:

➢ 1/2 Cup Butter, Melted

➢ 1 Package Chocolate Chip Cookie Mix

➢ 8-10 Drop Food Coloring

➢ 1/2 Tsp Mint, Extract

Directions:

1. Supply your smoker with wood pellets and follow the start-up procedure. Preheat the grill, with the lid closed, to 350° F.

2. Follow the directions on the back of the Chocolate Chip Cookie mix and also add the mint extract and green food coloring. Mix until combined.

3. On a baking sheet lined with parchment paper, drop balls of dough about 2 tbsp in size onto the pan.

4. Place in your Grill and bake for 10-12 minutes. Let cool for a couple minutes before removing from the pan. Enjoy!

Marbled Brownies With Amaretto & Ricotta

Servings: 4

Cooking Time: 30 Minutes

Ingredients:

- ➢ 1 Cup Ricotta Cheese
- ➢ 1 eggs
- ➢ 1 Tablespoon Amaretto Liqueur
- ➢ 1/4 Cup sugar
- ➢ 2 Teaspoon cornstarch
- ➢ 1/2 Teaspoon vanilla extract
- ➢ 1 Brownie Mix

Directions:

1. Coat a 9- by 13-inch nonstick baking pan with cooking spray or softened butter and set aside. (If you do not have a nonstick pan, line a regular one with buttered foil or parchment paper.)

2. In a medium bowl, combine the ricotta, egg, amaretto, sugar, cornstarch, and vanilla and whisk together thoroughly. Set aside.

3. Prepare the brownie mix according to the package directions. Spread the brownie batter evenly in the prepared pan. Randomly drop dollops of the ricotta mixture over the batter. Run a plastic knife through the ricotta mixture to give the brownies a marbled look. (A plastic knife is less likely to scratch your pan's nonstick surface.)

4. Supply your smoker with wood pellets and follow the start-up procedure. Preheat the grill, with the lid closed, to 350° F.

5. Put the pan with the brownie mixture directly on the grill grate and bake, about 25 to 30 minutes. Insert a bamboo skewer or toothpick in the center of the brownies to determine if they are done: the batter should not be wet. Grill: 350 °F

6. Transfer the brownies to a wire cooling rack to cool completely. Cut into squares.

Savory Beaver Tails

Servings: 8

Cooking Time: 2 Minutes

Ingredients:

- 2 Tbsp Butter, Melted
- 1 Tbsp Cinnamon, Ground
- 1 Egg
- 2 1/2 Cups Flour, All-Purpose
- 1/2 Cup Milk, Warm
- 1/2 Tsp Salt
- 1 Tsp Sugar
- 1/2 Tsp Vanilla
- 1 L Vegetable Oil
- 1/4 Cup Water, Warm
- 2 1/2 Tsp Active Yeast, Instant

Directions:

1. In a small bowl, combine water, milk, yeast, and sugar. Let it sit for about 10 minutes or until frothy.

2. In another bowl, pour in the flour and make a well in the middle. Pour in butter, sugar, salt, vanilla and egg. Mix everything together until the dough is smooth. Knead for about 5 minutes and set the dough in a greased bowl. Cover with a towel and set aside for about an hour, or until the dough has doubled in size.

3. After one hour, supply your smoker with wood pellets and follow the start-up procedure. Preheat the grill, with the lid open, to 450° F.Pour 1L of vegetable oil into a cast iron pan and place on the grates of your Grill. Keep your flame broiler closed so as to prevent grease flareups. Preheat the oil so that it is 350 degrees F.

4. While you"re waiting for the oil to heat up, punch down the dough and separate into 8 small balls. Shape each piece of dough into a flat circle. Fry the dough in the preheated oil for about 1 minute per side, or until the dough is golden brown.

5. Sprinkle with cinnamon sugar immediately, or top with your desired toppings. Enjoy!

Cinnamon Pull-aparts

Servings: 6

Cooking Time: 20 Minutes

Ingredients:

➢ 16.3 Ounce Biscuits, Homestyle, Canned

➢ 1 Cup packed brown sugar

➢ 1/2 Cup butter

➢ 1/4 Cup water

➢ 1 Teaspoon ground cinnamon

➢ 1/2 Cup Nuts (optional)

Directions:

1. Cut each biscuit into 4 pieces and peel each piece in half; set aside.

2. Combine brown sugar, butter and water in a large saucepan and bring to a boil; reduce heat and simmer for 1 minute. Stir in cinnamon and nuts; add biscuit quarters and mix to coat. Pour into greased 13 by 9 inch casserole dish and spread evenly in the dish.

3. Supply your smoker with wood pellets and follow the start-up procedure. Preheat the grill, with the lid closed, to 350° F.

4. Place the casserole dish on the grill; close lid and cook for 20 to 25 minutes or until the biscuits are done. Grill: 350 °F

5. Remove from the grill and transfer to a serving platter making sure to get all the gooey syrup onto the biscuits. Serve warm. Enjoy!

Chocolate Peanut Cookies

Servings: 4

Cooking Time: 12 Minutes

Ingredients:

- 1/2 Tsp Baking Soda
- 1/2 Cup Brown Sugar
- 1/2 Cup + 1 Tbsp Butter, Unsalted
- 1/3 Cup Cocoa Powder, Dark And Unsweetened
- 2 Eggs, Beaten
- 1 1/2 Cups Flour, All-Purpose
- 1/3 Cup Miniature Chocolate Chips
- 2 Cups Peanut Butter Chips, Divided
- 1/4 Tsp Sea Salt
- 1/2 Cup Sugar, Granulated
- 1 Tsp Vanilla Extract

Directions:

1. Supply your smoker with wood pellets and follow the start-up procedure. Preheat the grill, with the lid closed, to medium-low heat. If using a gas or charcoal grill, preheat a cast iron skillet.

2. In a mixing bowl, whisk together the flour, cocoa powder, baking soda, and salt. Set aside.

3. Set a metal saucepan on the griddle, then add ½ cup of butter to melt. Whisk in the sugars and vanilla extract and cook for 2 minutes. Remove the pan from the griddle, and transfer contents to a large mixing bowl.

4. Slowly pour the beaten eggs into the sugar mixture, whisking constantly to temper the eggs.

5. Add the dry mixture to the wet ingredients until just combined. Fold in 1 cup of peanut butter chips and chocolate chips. Refrigerate mixture for 15 to 30 minutes.

6. Remove the dough from the refrigerator, then add an additional cup of peanut butter chips.

7. Portion dough into 16 to 18 cookie balls.

8. Melt 1 tablespoon of butter on the griddle, then transfer the cookie balls to the griddle. Press down gently on the cookies, then cook for 10 to 12 minutes, flipping halfway.

9. Transfer cookies to a cooling rack for 5 minutes before enjoying.

Sopapilla Cheesecake By Doug Scheiding

Servings: 8

Cooking Time: 45 Minutes

Ingredients:

➢ 2 Tablespoon softened butter

➢ 24 Ounce cream cheese

➢ 2 Cup granulated sugar, divided

➢ 2 Teaspoon vanilla

➢ 2 Can Pillsbury Butter Flake Crescent Rolls

➢ 1/2 Cup butter, melted

➢ cinnamon

Directions:

1. Coat a 9x13 inch baking dish with 2 tablespoons softened butter and set aside.

2. Supply your smoker with wood pellets and follow the start-up procedure. Preheat the grill, with the lid closed, to 350° F.

3. In a mixer, combine cream cheese, 1 to 1-1/2 cups of sugar and vanilla. Mix for 60 to 90 seconds on high with paddle attachment.

4. Take crescents out of the refrigerator. Open one can and place into the buttered 9x13 inch rectangular metal pan or glass dish. Make sure to fill in the gaps in this bottom layer of crescents.

5. Put the cream cheese mixture on the top of the crescent layer using a spatula to make it level.

6. Open the second can of crescents and put on top of the cream cheese layer, again filling in the gaps in the crescents to cover middle.

7. Pour 1/2 cup of melted butter on the top of the last layer of crescent. Start on sides first then middle.

8. Then sprinkle 1/4 cup to 1/2 cup of sugar over the entire pan followed by a light, even dusting of cinnamon.

9. Place pan directly on the grill grate and bake for 40 to 50 minutes until top is brown and starting to get crusty. Grill: 350 °F

10. Remove from grill and let cool 5 to 10 minutes. This allows the cheesecake to set which makes portioning easier. This dessert can be served warm or cold. Enjoy!

Baked Bourbon Maple Pumpkin Pie

Servings: 6-8   Cooking Time: 60 Minutes

Ingredients:

- 1/4 Cup Cocoa Powder, Unsweetened
- 1 Tablespoon Cocoa Powder, Unsweetened
- 3 1/2 Tablespoon sugar
- 1 Teaspoon salt
- 1 1/4 Cup all-purpose flour
- 1 Tablespoon all-purpose flour
- 6 Tablespoon butter
- 2 Tablespoon vegetable oil
- 1 Large Egg Yolk
- 1/2 Teaspoon apple cider vinegar
- 1/4 Cup ice water
- 1 Large egg, beaten
- 15 Ounce Pumpkin, canned

- 1/4 Cup sour cream
- 2 Tablespoon bourbon
- 1 Teaspoon ground cinnamon
- 1/2 Teaspoon salt
- 1/4 Teaspoon ground ginger
- 1/4 Teaspoon ground nutmeg
- 1/8 Teaspoon Allspice, ground
- 1/8 Teaspoon Mace, ground
- 3 Large eggs
- 3/4 Cup maple syrup
- 2 Tablespoon sugar
- 1/2 Vanilla Bean, halved
- 1 Cup heavy cream

Directions:

1. For the Chocolate Pie Dough: Pulse cocoa powder, granulated sugar, salt, and 1-1/4 cups plus 1 Tbsp flour in a food processor to combine. Add butter and shortening and pulse until mixture resembles coarse meal with a few pea-sized pieces of butter remaining. Transfer to a large bowl.

2. Whisk together the egg yolk, vinegar, and 1/4 cup ice water in a small bowl. Drizzle half of the egg mixture over flour mixture and, using a fork, mix gently just until combined. Add remaining egg mixture and mix until the dough just comes together (you will have some unincorporated pieces).

3. Turn out dough onto a lightly floured surface, flatten slightly, and cut into quarters. Stack pieces on top of one another. Placing unincorporated dry pieces of dough between layers, and press down to combine. Repeat process twice more (all pieces of dough should be incorporated at this point). Form dough into a 1" thick disk. Wrap in plastic; chill at least 1 hour.

4. Roll out a disk of dough on a lightly floured surface into a 14" round. Transfer to a 9" pie dish. Lift up the edge and allow the dough to slump down into the dish. Trim. Leaving about 1" overhang. Fold overhang under and crimp edge. Chill in freezer 15 minutes.

5. When ready to cook, set the smoker to 350°F and preheat, lid closed for 15 minutes.

6. Line pie with parchment paper or heavy-duty foil, leaving a 1-1/2" overhang. Fill with pie weights or dried beans. Bake until crust is dry around the edge, about 20 minutes.

7. Remove paper and weights and bake until surface of the crust looks dry, 5-10 minutes.

8. Brush bottom and sides of crust with 1 beaten egg. Return to grill and bake until dry and set, about 3 minutes longer.

9. For the Pumpkin Maple Filling: Whisk together pumpkin puree, sour cream, bourbon, cinnamon, salt, ginger, nutmeg, allspice, mace (optional) and remaining 3 eggs in a large bowl; set aside.

10. Pour maple syrup and 2 tbsp sugar in a small saucepan. Scrape in the seeds from vanilla bean (reserve pod for another use) or add vanilla extract and bring syrup to a boil. Reduce heat to medium-high and simmer, stirring occasionally, until mixture is thickened and small puffs of steam start to release about 3 minutes.

11. Remove from heat and add cream in 3 additions, stirring with a wooden spoon after each addition until smooth. Gradually whisk hot maple cream into pumpkin mixture.

12. Place pie dish on a rimmed baking sheet and pour in pumpkin filling. Bake pie, rotating halfway through, until set around edge but center barely jiggles 50-60 minutes.

13. Transfer pie dish to a wire rack and let the pie cool. Slice and serve. Enjoy!

PORK RECIPES

Bacon Wrapped Pickles

Servings: 6

Cooking Time: 60 Minutes

Ingredients:

- ➢ 13 Strips Bacon
- ➢ 3 Bratwursts, Raw
- ➢ 1/2 Cup Colby Jack Cheese, Shredded
- ➢ 4 Oz Cream Cheese
- ➢ 13 Large Dill Pickles, Spears
- ➢ Hickory Bacon Rub
- ➢ 2 Scallion, Sliced Thin
- ➢ 1/4 Cup Sour Cream

Directions:

1. Supply your smoker with wood pellets and follow the start-up procedure. Preheat the grill, with the lid open, to 375° F.

2. Preheat griddle to medium- low flame.

3. In a mixing bowl combine cream cheese, sour cream, and scallions.

4. Use a hand mixer to blend well, then fold in grated cheddar-jack. Set aside.

5. Cook bratwurst on the griddle. Use a metal spatula to chop up sausage into smaller bits and cook until browned.

6. Remove from the griddle and set aside on a sheet tray to cool.

7. Place pickles on a sheet tray. Cut in half, then remove seeds with a small measuring spoon.

8. Stuff one half of each pickle with cream cheese mixture and top with crumbled bratwurst.

9. Top with the other pickle half, then wrap in bacon.

10. Season bacon-wrapped pickles with Hickory Bacon Rub, place in cast iron skillet, then transfer to grill.

11. Grill pickles for 45 to 55 minutes, until bacon starts to crisp on top. Remove from grill. Serve warm.

Simple Smoked Ribs

Servings: 6

Cooking Time: 240 Minutes

Ingredients:

➢ 3 Rack baby back ribs

➢ 3/4 Cup Pork & Poultry Rub

➢ 3/4 Cup 'Que BBQ Sauce

Directions:

1. Peel membrane from the back side of ribs and trim any excess fat.

2. Season both sides of ribs with Traeger Pork & Poultry Rub, about 1/4 cup per rack.

3. Supply your smoker with wood pellets and follow the start-up procedure. Preheat the grill, with the lid closed, to 180° F.

4. Place ribs on the grill and smoke for 3 to 4 hours. Grill: 180 °F Probe: 160 °F

5. When the internal temperature registers between 160°F to 165°F, remove ribs from the grill and increase Traeger temperature to 350°F. Grill: 350 °F

6. Place about 1/4 cup of Traeger 'Que BBQ Sauce on a large sheet of heavy-duty aluminum foil, then place a rack of ribs meat-side down on top and wrap tightly. Repeat with each rack.

7. Place the wrapped ribs back on the grill and cook for 45 minutes, or until internal temperature registers 204°F. Grill: 350 °F Probe: 204 °F

8. Remove from grill and let rest 20 minutes before slicing. Enjoy!

Stuffed Pork Crown Roast

Servings: 2-4   Cooking Time: 180 Minutes

Ingredients:

- 10 Pound Crown Roast of Pork, 12-14 ribs
- 1 Cup apple juice or cider
- 2 Tablespoon apple cider vinegar
- 2 Tablespoon Dijon mustard
- 1 Tablespoon brown sugar
- 2 Clove garlic, minced
- 2 Tablespoon Thyme or Rosemary, fresh
- 1 Teaspoon salt
- 1 Teaspoon coarse ground black pepper, divided
- 1/2 Cup olive oil
- 8 Cup Your Favorite Stuffing, Prepared According to the Package Directions, or Homemade

Directions:

1. Set the pork on a flat rack in a shallow roasting pan. Cover the end of each bone with a small piece of foil.

2. Make the marinade: Bring the apple cider to a boil over high heat and reduce by half. Remove from the heat, and whisk in the vinegar, mustard, brown sugar, garlic, thyme, and salt and pepper. Slowly whisk in the oil.

3. Using a pastry brush, apply the marinade to the roast, coating all surfaces. Cover it with plastic wrap and allow it to sit until the meat comes to room temperature, about 1 hour.

4. When ready to cook, set grill temperature to High and preheat, lid closed for 15 minutes.

5. Arrange the roasting pan with the pork on the grill grate. Roast for 30 minutes.

6. Reduce the heat to 325℉. Loosely fill the crown with the stuffing, mounding it at the top. Cover the stuffing with foil. (Alternatively, you can bake the stuffing in a separate pan alongside the roast.)

7. Roast the pork for another 1-1/2 hours. Remove the foil from the stuffing and continue to roast until the internal temperature of the meat is 150℉, about 30 minutes to an hour. Make sure the temperature probe doesn't touch bone or you will get a false reading.

8. Remove roast from grill and allow to rest for 15 minutes. Remove the foil covering the bones, but leave the butcher's string on the roast until ready to carve. Transfer to a warm platter.

9. To serve, carve between the bones. Enjoy!

St Louis Style Bbq Ribs With Texas Spicy Bbq Sauce

Servings: 8

Cooking Time: 300 Minutes

Ingredients:

➢ 3 Rack St. Louis-style ribs, membrane removed

➢ 4 Tablespoon Rub

➢ 6 Tablespoon butter

➢ 1 1/2 Cup brown sugar

➢ 1 1/2 Cup agave

➢ 1 1/2 Cup Texas Spicy BBQ Sauce

Directions:

1. Supply your smoker with wood pellets and follow the start-up procedure. Preheat the grill, with the lid closed, to 250° F.

2. Season ribs with Traeger rub and place directly on grill grate rib side down or in a Traeger rib rack with the bone resting on the rack. Cook for 3 hours. Grill: 250 ℉

3. Stack 2 pieces of tin foil on the table large enough to cover one rack of ribs. In the center of the foil place 3 tablespoons butter, 1/2 cup brown sugar, and 1/2 cup agave. Place the rib rack meat side down on top of the brown sugar mixture and wrap tightly. Repeat with remaining 2 racks.

4. Place all ribs directly on the grill grate meat side down and cook an additional 1-1/2 to 2 hours or until internal temperature reaches 203℉. Grill: 250 ℉ Probe: 203 ℉

5. Remove ribs from the grill and cover each rack with 1/2 cup Texas Spicy BBQ sauce.

6. Rewrap and return to grill an additional 10 minutes allowing sauce to thicken. Grill: 250 ℉

7. Remove ribs from the grill, slice and enjoy!

Pork Tenderloin With Bourbon Peaches

Servings: 6   Cooking Time: 27 Minutes

Ingredients:

- 2 pork tenderloins, about 2lb (1kg) total, trimmed of silver skin and excess fat
- extra virgin olive oil
- for the rub
- 3 tbsp coarse salt
- 3 tbsp freshly ground black pepper
- 3 tbsp smoked or regular paprika
- 3 tbsp granulated light brown sugar or low-carb substitute
- 2 tbsp instant coffee
- 1 tbsp granulated garlic
- 2 tsp ground cumin
- 1 tsp chili powder
- for the peaches
- 4 freestone peaches, about 1lb (450g) total, peeled, pitted, and sliced
- 1 tbsp freshly squeezed lemon juice
- ¼ cup unsalted butter
- 4 tbsp granulated light brown sugar or low-carb substitute
- 2 tbsp bourbon
- ½ tsp ground cinnamon
- ½ tsp pure vanilla extract
- pinch of coarse salt

Directions:

1. Supply your smoker with wood pellets and follow the start-up procedure. Preheat the grill, with the lid closed, to 400° F.

2. In a small bowl, make the rub by combining the ingredients. Coat the tenderloins in olive oil and season with the rub.

3. Place the peaches and lemon juice in a medium bowl, turning the peaches gently to coat. Measure the other ingredients and then take them and the peaches grill side.

4. Place 1 tablespoon of olive oil in the hot skillet and add the tenderloins. Quickly sear the pork, about 2 to 3 minute per side, turning as needed with tongs. When they're nicely browned, transfer the tenderloins to the grate. Cook until the internal temperature in the thickest part of the meat reaches 145°F (63°C), about 8 minutes. For moist meat, don't cook the tenderloins beyond 155°F (68°C).

5. Transfer the pork to a cutting board and tent with aluminum foil.

6. Replace the cast iron skillet with a clean one and close the grill lid to let it heat. Once hot, make the bourbon peaches by melting the butter. Add the brown sugar, bourbon, cinnamon, vanilla, and salt. Cook the mixture until it bubbles, about 5 to 8 minutes. Add the peaches and cook for 5 to 8 minutes more, turning the peaches carefully with a spoon to coat. Carefully transfer the skillet to a trivet or another heatproof surface.

7. Slice the pork on a diagonal into ½-inch (1.25cm) slices. Shingle the slices on a platter. Spoon the peaches around the pork or serve separately.

Red Onion Pork Butt With Sweet Chili Injection

Servings: 6   Cooking Time: 300 Minutes

Ingredients:

- To Taste, Blackened Sriracha Rub Seasoning
- 1/2 Tbsp Blackened Sriracha Rub Seasoning (For Injection)
- 1/4 Cup Butter, Melted
- 2 Cups Chicken Stock
- 1/2 Cup Chicken Stock (For Injection)
- 1 Tbsp Ginger Root, Sliced Thin
- 1/2 Lime, Juiced
- 1 Tbsp Olive Oil
- 5 Lbs Pork Butt, Bone-In
- 1 Red Onion, Sliced
- 1/4 Cup Rice Vinegar
- 1/2 Tbsp Sugar, Granulated
- 2 Tbsp Sweet Chili Sauce

Directions:

1. Place the pork butt on a sheet tray and pat dry with a paper towel.

2. Prepare the injection solution: Whisk together all ingredients in a glass measuring cup (1/2 cup Chicken Stock, 1/4 cup melted Butter, 1/4 cup Rice Wine Vinegar, 1/2 tbsp Blackened Sriracha Rub Seasoning, 1/2 Lime juice, 1/2 tbsp granulated Sugar).

3. Use a meat syringe to inject the solution into the pork butt, spacing every ½ inch.

4. Score the fat cap in a cross-hatch pattern, then rub sweet chili sauce on the outside of the pork butt, and season with Blackened Sriracha. Allow to sit at room temperature for 30 minutes.

5. Supply your smoker with wood pellets and follow the start-up procedure. Preheat the grill, with the lid open, to 250° F. If using a gas or charcoal grill, set it up for low, indirect heat.

6. Place the pork shoulder on the grill grate and smoke for 2 hours.

7. Place a Dutch oven or deep cast iron skillet on the grill. Heat olive oil, then add sliced onion and ginger, and set pork butt on top. Pour in chicken stock, then cover with a tight lid or foil.

8. Increase temperature to 325° F, and braise for 3 hours, until pork is tender. Remove the pork from the Dutch oven, and set aside to rest on a sheet tray, or cutting board.

9. Pull pork, then serve warm with braising jus.

Sweet Smoked Country Ribs

Servings: 12-15

Cooking Time: 240 Minutes

Ingredients:

- ➢ 2 pounds country-style ribs
- ➢ 1 batch Sweet Brown Sugar Rub
- ➢ 2 tablespoons light brown sugar
- ➢ 1 cup Pepsi or other cola
- ➢ ¼ cup The Ultimate BBQ Sauce

Directions:

1. Supply your smoker with wood pellets and follow the start-up procedure. Preheat the grill, with the lid closed, to 180°F.

2. Sprinkle the ribs with the rub and use your hands to work the rub into the meat.

3. Place the ribs directly on the grill grate and smoke for 3 hours.

4. Remove the ribs from the grill and place them on enough aluminum foil to wrap them completely. Dust the brown sugar over the ribs.

5. Increase the grill's temperature to 300°F.

6. Fold in three sides of the foil around the ribs and add the cola. Fold in the last side, completely enclosing the ribs and liquid. Return the ribs to the grill and cook for 45 minutes.

7. Remove the ribs from the foil and place them on the grill grate. Baste all sides of the ribs with barbecue sauce. Cook for 15 minutes more to caramelize the sauce.

8. Remove the ribs from the grill and serve immediately.

Smoked Bbq Ribs

Servings: 4

Cooking Time: 300 Minutes

Ingredients:

➢ 2 Rack St. Louis-style ribs

➢ 1/4 Cup Big Game Rub

➢ 1 Cup apple juice

➢ BBQ Sauce

Directions:

1. Pat ribs dry and peel the membrane from the back of the ribs.

2. Apply an even coat of rub to the front, back and sides of the ribs. Let sit for 20 minutes and up to 4 hours if refrigerated.

3. Supply your smoker with wood pellets and follow the start-up procedure. Preheat the grill, with the lid closed, to 225° F.

4. Place ribs, bone side down on grill. Put apple juice in a spray bottle and spray the ribs after 1 hour of cooking. Spray every 45 minutes thereafter. Grill: 225 °F Probe: 201 °F

5. After 4-1/2 hours, check the internal temperature of ribs. Ribs are done when internal temperature reaches 201°F. If not, check back in another 30 minutes. Grill: 225 °F Probe: 201 °F

6. Once ribs are done, brush a light layer of your favorite Traeger BBQ Sauce on the front and back of the ribs. Let the sauce set for 10 minutes. After the sauce has set, take ribs off the grill and let rest for 10 minutes. Slice ribs in between the bones and serve with extra sauce. Enjoy!

Competition Style Bbq Pork Ribs

Servings: 6

Cooking Time: 300 Minutes

Ingredients:

- ➢ 2 Rack St. Louis-style ribs
- ➢ 1 Cup Pork & Poultry Rub
- ➢ 1/8 Cup brown sugar
- ➢ 4 Tablespoon butter
- ➢ 4 Tablespoon agave
- ➢ 1 Bottle Sweet & Heat BBQ Sauce

Directions:

1. Supply your smoker with wood pellets and follow the start-up procedure. Preheat the grill, with the lid closed, to 225° F.

2. Remove membrane from back of ribs. Season with Traeger Pork & Poultry Rub on all sides. Let ribs rest for 15 to 20 minutes.

3. Place ribs on the grill, bone-side down and cook for 3 hours. While ribs are cooking, prepare the brown sugar wrap. Spread (approximately the same size as the rack of ribs) half the brown sugar, half the butter and half the agave on top of a double layer of aluminum foil. Repeat for second rack. Grill: 225 ℉

4. After 3 hours, place one rack of ribs meat side down in the brown sugar, butter and agave, and wrap. Repeat with second rack. Turn grill up to 250℉ and place wrapped ribs, meat side down in grill. Grill: 250 ℉

5. Cook for another 1-1/2 hours and check the internal temperature. Desired temperature is 204℉ to 205℉. If not at temperature, cook for an additional 30 minutes until temperature is reached. Grill: 250 ℉ Probe: 204 ℉

6. Remove ribs from the grill and foil packet. Place unwrapped ribs back in the grill for an additional 10 minutes. Remove from grill and sauce the meat and bone side with Traeger Sweet & Heat BBQ Sauce and cook for another 10 minutes. Slice ribs and serve. Enjoy!

Savory Pork Belly Banh Mi

Servings: 4   Cooking Time: 420 Minutes

Ingredients:

- 2 Carrots, Sliced
- 1 Tbsp Cilantro, Minced
- 1 Tbsp Honey
- 2 Kirby Cucumbers, Sliced Thin
- 1 Lime, Zest & Juice
- 2 Tbsp Pickling Spice
- 1 Tbsp Ponzu
- 2 Lbs Pork Belly
- 1 Cup Rice Wine Vinegar
- 2 Tbsp Salt
- 4 Sandwich Buns
- 1 Small Daikon Radish, Sliced Thin
- To Taste, Smoky Salt & Cracked Pepper Rub
- 2 Tbsp Soy Sauce
- 1/2 Cup Sriracha Hot Sauce
- 4 Cloves Star Anise
- 1/2 Cup Sugar
- 1 Cup Water

Directions:

1. 30 minutes before you plan to put the belly on the smoker season liberally with the Smoky Salt and Cracked Pepper rub.

2. Supply your smoker with wood pellets and follow the start-up procedure. Preheat the grill, with the lid open, to 240° F. If using a gas or charcoal grill, set it up for low, indirect heat.

3. Place the belly on the smoker with a tin pan underneath the meat to catch the drippings. Smoke for 7 hours or until you reach an internal temp of 195 degrees. Remove the pork and let rest for 30 minutes.

4. Make the homemade pickles: Place pickling spice and star anise in a small sauce pan and toast. Once fragrant add vinegar and bring to a boil, cook for 3 minutes. Add the water, sugar, and salt and return to a boil, cook for 5 minutes. Strain the liquid and immediately pour over the vegetables, making sure the vegetables are submerged. Set in the fridge once cool.

5. Make the Sriracha Lime Sauce: Combine the sriracha, lime, soy sauce, honey, cilantro and ponzu in a mixing bowl and whisk until combined.

6. Assemble the sandwiches, placing sliced pork belly and homemade pickles on a roll before topping it with the sriracha lime sauce.

Old-fashioned Roasted Glazed Ham

Servings: 8

Cooking Time: 60 Minutes

Ingredients:

- 1 (10 lb) fully cooked bone-in spiral cut ham
- 1 Cup pineapple juice
- 1/2 Cup brown sugar
- 1 cinnamon stick
- 14 whole cloves
- 1 Whole Pineapple, fresh
- 10 Cherries, fresh, sweet

Directions:

1. Supply your smoker with wood pellets and follow the start-up procedure. Preheat the grill, with the lid closed, to 325° F.

2. Rinse ham under cold water and pat dry with paper towel.

3. In a saucepan combine pineapple juice, brown sugar, cinnamon stick and four cloves. Bring to a boil. Reduce heat to medium low and simmer for about 15 minutes or until pineapple juice is reduced by half, thick and syrupy.

4. Brush half of the glaze onto the ham and into the folds of the cut slices. Reserve the other half of the glaze for later.

5. Cut pineapple in desired sized pieces, about 2 inch squares, then place on ham with a cherry and a clove to pin in place, repeating all over ham.

6. Put ham in a deep baking dish with fat side up. Place on the Traeger and cook for about 1-¼ hours. Grill: 325 °F

7. Carefully remove from Traeger and brush remaining glaze onto ham.

8. Return ham to Traeger and continue cooking for another 15 to 20 minutes, until internal temperature of ham reaches 160°F. Grill: 325 °F Probe: 160 °F

9. Allow ham to rest for 15 – 20 minutes before serving. Enjoy!

Unique Carolina Mustard Ribs

Servings: 4

Cooking Time: 300 Minutes

Ingredients:

➤ 1 Rack St. Louis Style Ribs

➤ 2 Cups Apple Juice

➤ 1/4 Cup Cider Vinegar

➤ 1/4 Cup Dark Brown Sugar

➤ 1/4 Cup Honey

➤ 1 Tablespoon Hot Sauce

➤ 2 Tablespoons Ketchup

➤ 7 Tablespoon Sweet Rib Rub

➤ 1 Tablespoon Worcestershire Sauce

➤ 2 Cups, Prepared Yellow Mustard

Directions:

1. Make the sauce for the ribs. In a large mixing bowl, combine 1 cup of the yellow mustard, cider vinegar, dark brown sugar, honey, ketchup, Worcestershire sauce, hot sauce, and 1 tablespoon of the Sweet Rib Rub. Mix well to combine and set in the refrigerator until ready to use.

2. Make the ribs. Using a paper towel, peel the membrane off of the backs of the rib racks and discard. Generously coat the ribs in a thin coat of mustard, and sprinkle all over with Sweet Rib Rub.

3. Supply your smoker with wood pellets and follow the start-up procedure. Preheat the grill, with the lid closed, to 275° F. If you're using a gas or charcoal grill set it up for low, indirect heat. Place the ribs meaty-side up and grill for 2-3 hours. Once the ribs have grilled for 2-3 hours, fill a spray bottle with 2 cups of apple juice and spray the ribs to keep them moist. Continue to grill the ribs, spraying every 45 minutes, until the meat bends slightly at the ends when lifted and is a deep mahogany color, about another 2-3 hours.

4. Remove the ribs from the grill and brush with mustard sauce, then slice and serve immediately.

SEAFOOD RECIPES

Peper Fish Tacos

Servings: 12

Cooking Time: 10 Minutes

Ingredients:

- ➢ 1 Tsp Black Pepper
- ➢ 1/4 Tsp Cayenne Pepper
- ➢ 1 1/2 Lbs Cod Fish
- ➢ 1/2 Tsp Cumin
- ➢ 1 Tsp Garlic Powder
- ➢ 1 Tsp Oregano
- ➢ 1 1/2 Tsp Paprika, Smoked
- ➢ 1/2 Tsp Salt

Directions:

1. Supply your smoker with wood pellets and follow the start-up procedure. Preheat the grill, with the lid closed, to 350° F.

2. Mix together paprika, garlic powder, oregano, cumin, cayenne, salt and pepper. Sprinkle over cod.

3. Place the cod on your preheated for about 5 minutes per side. Toast tortillas over heat, if desired.

4. Break the cod into pieces, smash the avocado, slice the tomatoes in half and place evenly among the tortillas. Top with red onion, lettuce, jalapenos, sour cream, and cilantro. Spritz with lime juice and enjoy!

Oysters In The Shell

Servings: 4

Cooking Time: 20 Minutes

Ingredients:

➢ 8 medium oysters, unopened, in the shell, rinsed and scrubbed

➢ 1 batch Lemon Butter Mop for Seafood

Directions:

1. Supply your smoker with wood pellets and follow the start-up procedure. Preheat the grill, with the lid closed, to 375°F.

2. Place the unopened oysters directly on the grill grate and grill for about 20 minutes, or until the oysters are done and their shells open.

3. Discard any oysters that do not open. Shuck the remaining oysters, transfer them to a bowl, and add the mop. Serve immediately.

Cedar Smoked Garlic Salmon

Servings: 6

Cooking Time: 60 Minutes

Ingredients:

- ➢ 1 Tsp Black Pepper
- ➢ 3 Cedar Plank, Untreated
- ➢ 1 Tsp Garlic, Minced
- ➢ 1/3 Cup Olive Oil
- ➢ 1 Tsp Onion, Salt
- ➢ 1 Tsp Parsley, Minced Fresh
- ➢ 1 1/2 Tbsp Rice Vinegar
- ➢ 2 Salmon, Fillets (Skin Removed)
- ➢ 1 Tsp Sesame Oil
- ➢ 1/3 Cup Soy Sauce

Directions:

1. Soak the cedar planks in warm water for an hour or more.
2. In a bowl, mix together the olive oil, rice vinegar, sesame oil, soy sauce, and minced garlic.
3. Add in the salmon and let it marinate for about 30 minutes.
4. Start your grill on smoke with the lid open until a fire is established in the burn pot (3-7 minutes).
5. Supply your smoker with wood pellets and follow the start-up procedure. Preheat the grill, with the lid closed, to 225° F.
6. Place the planks on the grate. Once the boards start to smoke and crackle a little, it's ready for the fish.
7. Remove the fish from the marinade, season it with the onion powder, parsley and black pepper, then discard the marinade.
8. Place the salmon on the planks and grill until it reaches 140°F internal temperature (start checking temp after the salmon has been on the grill for 30 minutes).
9. Remove from the grill, let it rest for 10 minutes, then serve.

Smoked Salmon Candy

Servings: 4

Cooking Time: 180 Minutes

Ingredients:

- ➢ 2 Cup gin
- ➢ 1 Cup dark brown sugar
- ➢ 1/2 Cup kosher salt
- ➢ 1 Cup maple syrup
- ➢ 1 Tablespoon black pepper
- ➢ 3 Pound salmon
- ➢ vegetable oil
- ➢ dark brown sugar

Directions:

1. In a large bowl, combine all ingredients for the cure.
2. Cut the salmon into 2 ounce pieces and place in the cure.
3. Cover and refrigerate overnight.
4. Supply your smoker with wood pellets and follow the start-up procedure. Preheat the grill, with the lid closed, to 180° F.
5. Spray foil with vegetable oil. Place salmon on foil and sprinkle with additional brown sugar.
6. Place foil directly on the grill grate. Close the lid and smoke the salmon for 3 to 4 hours or until fully cooked. Grill: 180 °F
7. Serve hot or chilled. Enjoy!

Baked Tuna Noodle Casserole

Servings: 4

Cooking Time: 45 Minutes

Ingredients:

➢ 1 Whole Wheat Pasta, Box (13.25oz)

➢ 2 Cup Yogurt

➢ 1 Cup almond milk

➢ 1 Teaspoon ground mustard

➢ 1/2 Teaspoon celery salt

➢ 1 Cup Button Mushrooms, Sliced

➢ 10 Ounce Tuna, Cooked

➢ 1 Cup Peas, canned

➢ 1 Cup Cheese, Colby/Cheddar

Directions:

1. Bring a large pot of salted water to a boil over high heat. Add pasta and cook according to manufacturer's directions. Drain and set aside.

2. In a medium bowl mix yogurt, milk, ground mustard, and celery salt. Fold in mushrooms, tuna, peas and cooked pasta. Fold in half the cheese.

3. Transfer the mixture to a greased 13" x 9" baking dish and top with remaining cheese.

4. Supply your smoker with wood pellets and follow the start-up procedure. Preheat the grill, with the lid closed, to 350° F.

5. Place casserole dish directly on grill grate and cook for 45 minutes or until warmed through and cheese is melted. Enjoy! Grill: 350 °F

Spicy Shrimp Skewers

Servings: 4

Cooking Time: 6 Minutes

Ingredients:

- ➢ 2 Pound shrimp, peeled and deveined
- ➢ 6 Thai chiles
- ➢ 6 Clove garlic
- ➢ 2 Tablespoon Winemaker's Napa Valley Rub
- ➢ 1 1/2 Teaspoon sugar
- ➢ 1 1/2 Tablespoon white vinegar
- ➢ 3 Tablespoon olive oil

Directions:

1. If using bamboo skewers, place them in cold water to soak for 1 hour before grilling.

2. Place shrimp in a bowl and set aside. Combine all remaining ingredients in a blender and blend until a coarse-textured paste is reached. Note: if a milder flavor is preferred, feel free to adjust amount of chiles to taste.

3. Add chile-garlic mixture to the shrimp and place in fridge to marinate for at least 30 minutes.

4. Remove from fridge and thread shrimp onto bamboo or metal skewers.

5. Supply your smoker with wood pellets and follow the start-up procedure. Preheat the grill, with the lid closed, to 450° F.

6. Place shrimp on grill and cook for 2 to 3 minutes per side or until shrimp are pink and firm to touch. Enjoy! Grill: 450 ˚F

Pacific Northwest Salmon

Servings: 4

Cooking Time: 75 Minutes

Ingredients:

➢ 1 (2-pound) half salmon fillet

➢ 1 batch Dill Seafood Rub

➢ 2 tablespoons butter, cut into 3 or 4 slices

Directions:

1. Supply your smoker with wood pellets and follow the start-up procedure. Preheat the grill, with the lid closed, to 180°F.

2. Season the salmon all over with the rub. Using your hands, work the rub into the flesh.

3. Place the salmon directly on the grill grate, skin-side down, and smoke for 1 hour.

4. Place the butter slices on the salmon, equally spaced. Increase the grill's temperature to 300°F and continue to cook until the salmon's internal temperature reaches 145°F. Remove the salmon from the grill and serve immediately.

Lime Mahi Mahi Fillets

Servings: 4

Cooking Time: 8 Minutes

Ingredients:

- ➢ 3/4 cup extra-virgin olive oil
- ➢ 1 clove garlic, minced
- ➢ 1/8 teaspoon ground black pepper
- ➢ 1/2 teaspoon cayenne pepper
- ➢ 2 tablespoons dill weed.
- ➢ 1 pinch salt
- ➢ 2 tablespoons lime juice
- ➢ 1/8 teaspoon grated lime peel
- ➢ 2 (4 ounce) mahi mahi fillets

Directions:

1. Supply your smoker with wood pellets and follow the start-up procedure. Preheat the grill, with the lid closed, to 325° F.

2. Lightly oil the grate.

3. Combine in a bowl the extra-virgin olive oil, minced garlic, black pepper, cayenne pepper, salt, lime juice, and grated lime zest.

4. Wisk to prepare the marinade.

5. Place the mahi mahi fillets in the marinade and turn to coat.

6. Allow to marinate at least 15 minutes.

7. Cook on preheated grill until fish flakes easily with a fork and is lightly browned (Typically 3 to 4 minutes per side).

8. Garnish with the twists of lime zest to serve.

Cold-smoked Salmon Gravlax

Servings: 6

Cooking Time: 30 Minutes

Ingredients:

- 1 Cup kosher salt
- 1 Cup sugar
- 1 Tablespoon freshly ground black pepper
- 2 Pound Sushi-Grad Salmon Fillet, Skin-on, Pin Bones Removed
- 2 Bunch Dill Weed, fresh
- capers, drained
- red onion, sliced
- cream cheese
- lemons

Directions:

1. In a bowl stir together the salt, sugar and black pepper until thoroughly combined. On a work surface, turn salmon skin side up and sprinkle about half of salt mixture all over and rub in.

2. Arrange half the dill on the bottom of a baking dish large enough to hold the salmon. Set salmon skin side down on bed of dill.

3. Rub remaining salt mixture all over top and sides of salmon, then top with remaining dill. Cover with plastic, then top with a weight on a smaller baking dish or a plate with cans of beans on top, then place in refrigerator and allow to cure for 2 days.

4. Remove salmon from refrigerator, rinse under cold water and pat dry with paper towels. Allow to sit at room temperature on the counter for 1 hour

5. Supply your smoker with wood pellets and follow the start-up procedure. Preheat the grill, with the lid closed, to 180° F. Place salmon onto a baking pan. Fill another baking pan with ice and place baking pan with salmon over ice. Place onto grill and smoke for 30 minutes.

6. Remove from grill and slice thin. Serve with capers, red onion, dill, cream cheese, and lemon. Enjoy!

Grilled Albacore Tuna With Potato-tomato Casserole

Servings: 8

Cooking Time: 20 Minutes

Ingredients:

- ➢ 6 Tuna Steaks, 6oz
- ➢ 1 Whole lemon zest
- ➢ 1 chile de árbol, thinly sliced
- ➢ 1 Tablespoon thyme
- ➢ 1 Tablespoon fresh parsley

Directions:

1. To make the fish: Season the fish with the lemon zest, chile, thyme, and parsley. Cover and refrigerate at least 4 hours.

2. Remove fish from the refrigerator 30 minutes before cooking to come to room temperature.

3. Season the fish with salt and pepper on both sides. Grill 2-3 minutes per side (next to the cast iron with the casserole) rotating it once or twice. The tuna should be well seared but still rare.

Smoked Fish Chowder

Servings: 4

Cooking Time: 60 Minutes

Ingredients:

➢ 12 Ounce (1-1/2 to 2 lb) skin-on salmon fillet, preferably wild-caught
➢ Fin & Feather Rub
➢ 2 Corn Husks
➢ 3 Slices Bacon, sliced
➢ 4 Can Cream of Potato Soup, Condensed
➢ 3 Cup whole milk
➢ 8 Ounce cream cheese
➢ 3 green onions, thinly sliced
➢ 2 Teaspoon hot sauce

Directions:

1. Supply your smoker with wood pellets and follow the start-up procedure. Preheat the grill, with the lid closed, to 180° F.

2. Sprinkle Traeger Fin & Feather rub as needed on salmon. Arrange the salmon skin-side down on the grill grate. Smoke for 30 minutes. Grill: 180 ℉

3. Increase the grill temperature to 350℉. Grill: 350 ℉

4. Cook the salmon for 30 minutes, or until the fish flakes easily with a fork. (The exact time will depend on the thickness of the fillet.) There is no need to turn the fish. Using a large thin spatula, transfer the salmon to a wire rack to cool. Remove the skin. (The salmon can be made a day ahead, wrapped in plastic wrap and refrigerated.) Break into flakes and set aside.

5. Arrange the corn and bacon strips on the grill grate. (The salmon will be roasting while you do this.) Roast the corn and the bacon until the corn is cooked through and browned in spots, turning as needed, and the bacon is crisp, about 15 minutes.

6. In the meantime, bring the cream of potato soup and the milk to a simmer over medium heat in a large saucepan or Dutch oven on the stovetop. Gradually stir in the cream cheese and whisk to blend. Chop the bacon into bits and slice the corn off the cobs using long strokes of a chef's knife.

7. Add to the soup along with the green onions. Stir in the salmon. Heat gently for 5 to 10 minutes. Add the hot sauce to taste. If the chowder is too thick, add more milk. Serve at once. Enjoy!

Prosciutto-wrapped Scallops

Servings: 4

Cooking Time: 10 Minutes

Ingredients:

- ➢ 1½lb (680g) jumbo sea or diver scallops (size U-10)
- ➢ 8 to 10 thin slices of prosciutto, each halved lengthwise
- ➢ coarse salt
- ➢ freshly ground black pepper
- ➢ for the butter
- ➢ 8oz (225g) unsalted butter
- ➢ 2 tsp minced fresh curly or flat-leaf parsley
- ➢ 1½ tsp finely grated orange zest
- ➢ 1 tbsp freshly squeezed orange juice
- ➢ 1 tsp finely grated lemon zest
- ➢ 1 tsp finely grated lime zest
- ➢ ½ tsp coarse salt

Directions:

1. Supply your smoker with wood pellets and follow the start-up procedure. Preheat the grill, with the lid closed, to 450° F.

2. In a small saucepan on the stovetop over medium-low heat, make the citrus butter by melting the butter. Add the remaining ingredients and simmer for 3 to 5 minutes to blend the flavors. Keep warm.

3. Rinse the scallops under cold running water and dry with paper towels. Place each scallop on its side at the end of a piece of prosciutto and wrap the prosciutto around the scallop. Secure with a toothpick. Season the exposed sides of the scallop with salt and pepper.

4. Place the scallops exposed sides down on the grate and grill until the edges of the prosciutto begin to frizzle and the scallop is warm inside, about 3 to 5 minutes per side.

5. Transfer the scallops to a platter. Brush with some of the warm citrus butter before serving. Serve the remaining butter on the side.

POULTRY RECIPES

Asian Bbq Chicken

Servings: 4

Cooking Time: 60 Minutes

Ingredients:

➤ 1 Whole whole chicken

➤ Asian BBQ Rub

➤ 1 Whole ginger ale

Directions:

1. Rinse chicken in cold water and pat dry with paper towels. Cover the chicken all over with Traeger Asian BBQ rub; make sure to drop some in the inside too. Place in large bag or bowl and cover and refrigerate for 12 to 24 hours.

2. Supply your smoker with wood pellets and follow the start-up procedure. Preheat the grill, with the lid closed, to 375° F.

3. Open your can of ginger ale and take a few big gulps. Set the can of soda on a stable surface. Take the chicken out of the fridge and place the bird over top of the soda can. The base of the can and the two legs of the chicken should form a sort of tripod to hold the chicken upright.

4. Stand the chicken in the center of your hot grate and cook the chicken till the skin is golden brown and the internal temperature is about 165°F on a instant-read thermometer, approximately 40 minutes to 1 hour.

5. De-throne chicken. Enjoy!

Smoked Chicken Fajita Quesadillas

Servings: 4

Cooking Time: 45 Minutes

Ingredients:

- 2 Chicken, Boneless/Skinless
- 1 Tsp Chilli, Powder
- 1 Tsp Garlic Powder
- 1/2 Green Bell Pepper, Sliced
- 1 Cup Mexican Cheese, Shredded
- 1/2 Onion, Sliced
- 1/2 Tsp Oregano
- 1 Tsp Paprika, Powder
- 1/4 Tsp Pepper
- 1/2 Red Bell Peppers
- Salsa
- Sour Cream
- 4 Tortilla
- 1/2 Yellow Bell Pepper, Sliced

Directions:

1. Supply your smoker with wood pellets and follow the start-up procedure. Preheat the grill, with the lid open, to 350° F.

2. Combine spices in a bowl and season chicken breasts. Leave a little bit of seasoning for the vegetables.

3. Place chicken on the grates and cook for 30 minutes, flipped halfway through.

4. In a Vegetable Basket, combine all vegetables and season with the remaining spice mixture.

5. Open up the flame broiler and saute over the open flame for about 15 minutes, or until the vegetables are cooked to your liking.

6. On a tortilla, layer cheese, vegetables, sliced chicken and more cheese. Fold the tortilla and place over the open flame on your Grill. Sear until the tortilla is nicely toasted and the cheese is melted. Cut and serve with salsa and sour cream.

Grilled Honey Chicken Kabobs

Servings: 4

Cooking Time: 14 Minutes

Ingredients:

- 1 pound boneless skinless chicken breasts (cut into 1 inch pieces)
- 1/4 cup olive oil
- 1/3 cup soy sauce
- 1/4 cup honey
- 1 teaspoon minced garlic
- salt and pepper to taste
- 1 red bell pepper (cut into 1 inch pieces)
- 1 yellow bell pepper (cut into 1 inch pieces)
- 2 small zucchini (cut into 1 inch slices)
- 1 red onion (cut into 1 inch pieces)
- 1 tablespoon chopped parsley

Directions:

1. In a large bowl combine the olive oil, soy sauce, honey, garlic and salt and pepper, and whisk.
2. Add the chicken, bell peppers, zucchini and red onion to the bowl, tossing to thoroughly coat.
3. Cover and refrigerate for 1 to 8 hours.
4. Soak wooden skewers in cold water for at least 30 minutes. Supply your smoker with wood pellets and follow the start-up procedure. Preheat the grill, with the lid closed, to high heat.
5. Thread the chicken and vegetables onto the skewers.
6. Cook for 5-7 minutes on each side or until chicken is cooked through.
7. To serve, sprinkle with parsley. Enjoy!

Chicken Egg Rolls With Buffalo Sauce

Servings: 4   Cooking Time: 75 Minutes

Ingredients:

- 1/4 Cup Bleu Cheese, Crumbled
- 1/4 Cup Buffalo Sauce
- 1 Lb Chicken Breasts - Boneless, Skinless
- 4 Oz Cream Cheese, Softened
- 8 Egg Roll Wrappers
- 1/2 Jalapeno Pepper, Minced

- Pinch Sweet Heat Rub
- 1/4 Red Bell Pepper, Chopped
- 4 Scallion, Sliced Thin
- 1/4 Cup Sour Cream
- 2 Cups Vegetable Oil

Directions:

1. Supply your smoker with wood pellets and follow the start-up procedure. Preheat the grill, with the lid open, to 200° F. If using a gas or charcoal grill, set it up for low, indirect heat.

2. Season chicken breasts with   Sweet Heat Rub, then place on the grill. Smoke for 1 hour, then remove from the grill, cool, shred, and set aside.

3. Prepare the filling: In a mixing bowl, use a hand mixer to blend cream cheese, bleu cheese, Buffalo sauce and sour cream.

4. Fold in scallions, jalapeño, red bell pepper, and shredded chicken.

5. Prepare egg rolls: Lay an egg roll wrapper on a flat surface and add 3 tablespoons of filling to the middle.

6. Fold the bottom of the wrapper over the top of the filling, then fold over each side. Brush the top point of the wrapper with warm water, then roll the wrapper tight. Transfer to a tray while filling the remaining wrappers.

7. Increase the temperature of the grill to 425°F, then set a cast iron Dutch oven on the grill. Add vegetable oil and heat for 5 minutes.

8. Place 3 egg rolls in heated oil and fry until golden, 1 to 2 minutes per side.

9. Transfer to a wire rack to cool, then fry the remaining egg rolls, in batches.

10. Cool egg rolls for 2 minutes, then slice in half and serve warm with celery sticks and extra Buffalo sauce for dipping.

Grilled Greek Chicken With Garlic & Lemon

Servings: 4

Cooking Time: 60 Minutes

Ingredients:

➤ 2 Whole Roasting Chicken, 3.5-4lbs, each cut into 8 pieces

➤ 2 Whole lemons, quartered

➤ Cup extra-virgin olive oil

➤ 4 Clove garlic, minced

➤ 1 1/2 Tablespoon Oregano, fresh

➤ 1 As Needed Chicken Rub

➤ 1 Cup Broth, chicken

Directions:

1. Arrange the chicken pieces in a single layer in a large roasting pan. Squeeze the juice from each piece of lemon over the chicken, catching any seeds in your fingers. Tuck the lemon rinds in with the chicken. Drizzle the olive oil over all.

2. Sprinkle the garlic over the chicken. Dust the chicken with the fresh oregano, and season it generously with the Traeger Chicken rub, or salt and black pepper. Pour the chicken broth into the pan.

3. Supply your smoker with wood pellets and follow the start-up procedure. Preheat the grill, with the lid closed, to 350° F.

4. Roast the chicken for an hour, or until the juices run clear or the internal temperature reaches 165°F on an instant-read meat thermometer. Grill: 350 °F Probe: 165 °F

5. Transfer to a platter or plates and spoon some of the juices on top. Let rest 3 minutes before serving. Enjoy!

Smoked Quarters

Servings: 2-4

Cooking Time: 120 Minutes

Ingredients:

- ➢ 4 chicken quarters
- ➢ 2 tablespoons olive oil
- ➢ 1 batch Chicken Rub
- ➢ 2 tablespoons butter

Directions:

1. Supply your smoker with wood pellets and follow the start-up procedure. Preheat the grill, with the lid closed, to 180°F.

2. Coat the chicken quarters all over with olive oil and season them with the rub. Using your hands, work the rub into the meat.

3. Place the quarters directly on the grill grate and smoke for 1½ hours.

4. Baste the quarters with the butter and increase the grill's temperature to 375°F. Continue to cook until the chicken's internal temperature reaches 170°F.

5. Remove the quarters from the grill and let them rest for 10 minutes before serving.

Wild West Wings

Servings: 4

Cooking Time: 60 Minutes

Ingredients:

- ➤ 2 pounds chicken wings
- ➤ 2 tablespoons extra-virgin olive oil
- ➤ 2 packages ranch dressing mix (such as Hidden Valley brand)
- ➤ ¼ cup prepared ranch dressing (optional)

Directions:

1. Supply your smoker with wood pellets and follow the start-up procedure. Preheat, with the lid closed, to 350°F.

2. Place the chicken wings in a large bowl and toss with the olive oil and ranch dressing mix.

3. Arrange the wings directly on the grill, or line the grill with aluminum foil for easy cleanup, close the lid, and smoke for 25 minutes.

4. Flip and smoke for 20 to 35 minutes more, or until a meat thermometer inserted in the thickest part of the wings reads 165°F and the wings are crispy. (Note: The wings will likely be done after 45 minutes, but an extra 10 to 15 minutes makes them crispy without drying the meat.)

5. Serve warm with ranch dressing (if using).

Smoked Whole Chicken

Servings: 6-8

Cooking Time: 240 Minutes

Ingredients:

➢ 1 whole chicken

➢ 2 cups Tea Injectable (using Not-Just-for-Pork Rub)

➢ 2 tablespoons olive oil

➢ 1 batch Chicken Rub

➢ 2 tablespoons butter, melted

Directions:

1. Supply your smoker with wood pellets and follow the start-up procedure. Preheat the grill, with the lid closed, to 180°F.

2. Inject the chicken throughout with the tea injectable.

3. Coat the chicken all over with olive oil and season it with the rub. Using your hands, work the rub into the meat.

4. Place the chicken directly on the grill grate and smoke for 3 hours.

5. Baste the chicken with the butter and increase the grill's temperature to 375°F. Continue to cook the chicken until its internal temperature reaches 170°F.

6. Remove the chicken from the grill and let it rest for 10 minutes, before carving and serving.

Buffalo Chicken Thighs

Servings: 4

Cooking Time: 15 Minutes

Ingredients:

- 6 bone-in, skin-on chicken thighs
- Pork & Poultry Rub
- 2 Cup Buffalo wing sauce
- 8 Tablespoon butter
- blue cheese crumbles, for serving
- ranch dressing, for serving

Directions:

1. Supply your smoker with wood pellets and follow the start-up procedure. Preheat the grill, with the lid closed, to 450° F.

2. Generously season the chicken thighs with Traeger Pork & Poultry Rub and place directly on the grill grate. Grill: 450 °F

3. Cook for 8 to 10 minutes, flipping once. Grill: 450 °F

4. In a small saucepan, combine the wing sauce and the butter over medium heat, stirring occasionally.

5. Dip the cooked chicken thighs into the wing sauce and butter mixture, turning to coat both sides evenly. Grill: 450 °F Probe: 175 °F

6. Return the sauced chicken thighs to the grill and cook for an additional 4 to 5 minutes, or until the internal temperature reads 175°F on an instant-read meat thermometer. Grill: 450 °F Probe: 175 °F

7. Sprinkle with the blue cheese and drizzle with ranch dressing, if desired. Enjoy!

Turkey & Bacon Kebabs With Ranch-style Dressing

Servings: 8   Cooking Time: 25 Minutes

Ingredients:

- 1½lb (680g) skinless turkey tenders or boneless, skinless turkey breasts, cut into 1-inch (2.5cm) chunks
- 8 strips of thick-cut bacon
- 12 fresh bay leaves (optional)
- for the dressing
- 1 cup reduced-fat mayo
- 1 cup light sour cream
- ½ cup buttermilk or whole milk, plus more
- 2 tbsp minced fresh parsley
- 2 tbsp minced fresh chives
- 1 tbsp minced fresh dill
- 2 tsp freshly squeezed lemon juice
- 1 tsp Worcestershire sauce
- 1 tsp garlic salt
- 1 tsp onion powder
- ½ tsp coarse salt, plus more
- ½ tsp freshly ground black pepper, plus more

Directions:

1. In a large bowl, make the dressing by whisking together the mayo, sour cream, and buttermilk until smooth. Whisk in the remaining ingredients. Pour half the mixture into a small bowl. Cover and refrigerate.

2. Add the turkey to the mixture remaining in the bowl and toss to coat thoroughly. If the dressing seems too thick (dip-like), add more buttermilk 1 tablespoon at a time. Cover and refrigerate for 2 to 4 hours.

3. Supply your smoker with wood pellets and follow the start-up procedure. Preheat the grill, with the lid closed, to 375° F.

4. Place the bacon on the grate and cook until some of the fat has rendered and the bacon begins to brown, about 15 minutes. Remove the bacon from the grill to cool. Cut the bacon into 1-inch (2.5cm) squares. Set aside.

5. Drain the tenders and discard any excess dressing. Alternate threading the turkey, bacon pieces, and 3 bay leaves on a bamboo skewer. Repeat the threading with 3 more skewers.

6. Place the kebabs on the grate and grill until the turkey is cooked through, about 4 to 5 minutes per side, turning as needed.

7. Transfer the skewers to a platter. Serve with the reserved dressing.

Juicy Jerk Chicken Kebabs

Servings: 4

Cooking Time: 12 Minutes

Ingredients:

- 1 Tablespoon All Spice, Ground
- 2 Lbs Chicken, Boneless/Skinless
- 1 Tablespoon Cinnamon, Ground
- 1/4 Cup Extra-Virgin Olive Oil
- 3 Garlic, Cloves
- 2 Inch Piece Ginger, Fresh
- 3 Green Onion
- 1 Lime, Juiced
- 1 Tablespoon Nutmeg, Ground
- 1 Cup Orange Juice, Fresh
- Pepper
- 1 Red Onion, Chopped
- Salt
- Skewers
- 1/4 Cup Soy Sauce
- 1/4 Cup Thyme, Fresh Sprigs

Directions:

1. Soak the bamboo skewers in water for about 30 minutes (the longer the better).

2. In a food processor, combine orange juice, oil, soy sauce, thyme, allspice, nutmeg, cinnamon, garlic, onions, ginger, lime juice, salt and pepper. Puree until smooth.

3. In a large resealable bag, pour all but 1/4 cup of the mixture in along with the sliced up chicken breasts. Seal the bag and marinate in the fridge for 2 - 3 hours.

4. Supply your smoker with wood pellets and follow the start-up procedure. Preheat the grill, with the lid open, to 450° F. Skewer the chicken and grill for about 7 minutes. Flip and continue grilling for about 5 minutes, or until the chicken is cooked through and grill marks appear. Serve with the remaining 1/4 cup of marinade.

Peanut Butter Chicken Wings

Servings: 4

Cooking Time: 35 Minutes

Ingredients:

➢ 1 Tsp Black Peppercorns, Ground

➢ 2 Tbsp Brown Sugar

➢ 4 Lbs Chicken Wings, Trimmed And Patted Dry

➢ 2 Tbsp Honey

➢ 1/4 Cup Peanut Butter

➢ 10 Oz Peanuts, Whole

➢ 2 Tsp Sweet Rib Rub

➢ 1/2 Red Onion, Minced

➢ 1/2 Cup Strawberry Preserves

➢ 1 Tbsp Thai Chili Sauce

➢ 1/4 Cup Worcestershire Sauce

Directions:

1. Place chicken wings in a 9 x13 glass baking dish. Pour mixture over chicken, cover with plastic wrap, and refrigerate for 2 hours.

2. Supply your smoker with wood pellets and follow the start-up procedure. Preheat the grill, with the lid open, to 400° F. Preheat griddle to medium-low flame. If using a gas or charcoal grill, set it to medium-high heat.

3. Place wings directly on grill grate, over indirect heat, and cook for 20 to 25 minutes, rotating wings every 5 minutes.

4. Meanwhile, place shelled peanuts on the griddle, turning occasionally with a metal spatula for 5 to 7 minutes, to lightly roast. Remove from the griddle and set aside to cool.

5. Remove wings from grill and allow to rest for 5 minutes. While wings are resting, shell the peanuts, and transfer to a resealable plastic bag. Use a rolling pin to crush the peanuts, then scatter peanuts on top of the chicken wings. Serve warm.

VEGETABLES RECIPES

Mashed Red Potatoes

Servings: 4

Cooking Time: 40 Minutes

Ingredients:

➢ 8 Large red potatoes

➢ salt

➢ black pepper

➢ 1/2 Cup heavy cream

➢ 1/4 Cup butter

Directions:

1. Supply your smoker with wood pellets and follow the start-up procedure. Preheat the grill, with the lid closed, to 180° F.

2. Slice red potatoes in half, lengthwise then cut in half again to make quarters. Season potatoes with salt and pepper.

3. Increase the heat to High and preheat. Once the grill is hot, set potatoes directly on the grill grate. Grill: 450 °F

4. Every 15 minutes flip potatoes to ensure all sides get color. Continue to do this until potatoes are fork tender.

5. When tender, mash potatoes with cream, butter, salt, and pepper to taste. Serve warm, enjoy!

Baked Kale Chips

Servings: 4

Cooking Time: 20 Minutes

Ingredients:

➢ 2 Bunch kale, leaves washed and stems removed

➢ 1 As Needed extra-virgin olive oil

➢ 1 To Taste sea salt

Directions:

1. Dry the kale leaves well and lay them out on a sheet tray. Drizzle lightly with olive oil and sprinkle with sea salt.

2. Supply your smoker with wood pellets and follow the start-up procedure. Preheat the grill, with the lid closed, to 250° F.

3. Place the sheet tray directly on the grill grate and cook until kale is lightly browned and crispy, about 20 minutes. Enjoy! Grill: 250 ˚F

Portobello Marinated Mushroom

Servings: 2

Cooking Time: 15 Minutes

Ingredients:

- ➢ 1 Teaspoon chopped thyme
- ➢ 1 Teaspoon rosemary, chopped
- ➢ 1 Teaspoon Oregano, chopped
- ➢ 3 Tablespoon extra-virgin olive oil
- ➢ 1 To Taste Jacobsen Salt Co. Pure Kosher Sea Salt
- ➢ 1 To Taste pepper
- ➢ 6 Whole Portobello Mushroom
- ➢ 2 Whole russet potatoes

Directions:

1. Supply your smoker with wood pellets and follow the start-up procedure. Preheat the grill, with the lid closed, to 450° F.

2. Mix fresh herbs, olive oil, salt, and pepper together in a bowl. Rub over mushrooms. Grill both sides of mushrooms for approximately 2-3 minutes on each side. Grill: 450 ˚F

3. Clean the potatoes and slice into long strips.

4. Heat the oil on the Traeger in a sauce pan; drop the potatoes in the hot oil and fry for 7-8 minutes. Let the potatoes cool slightly on a sheet pan. Enjoy! Grill: 450 ˚F

Roasted Asparagus

Servings: 4

Cooking Time: 30 Minutes

Ingredients:

➢ 1 Bunch asparagus

➢ 2 Tablespoon olive oil, plus more as needed

➢ Veggie Rub

Directions:

1. Coat asparagus with olive oil and Veggie Rub, stirring to coat all pieces.

2. Supply your smoker with wood pellets and follow the start-up procedure. Preheat the grill, with the lid closed, to 350° F.

3. Place asparagus directly on the grill grate for 15-20 minutes.

4. Remove from grill and enjoy!

Roasted Green Beans With Bacon

Servings: 4

Cooking Time: 20 Minutes

Ingredients:

- ➢ 1 1/2 Pound green beans, ends trimmed
- ➢ 4 Strips bacon, cut into small pieces
- ➢ 4 Tablespoon extra-virgin olive oil
- ➢ 2 Clove garlic, minced
- ➢ 1 Teaspoon kosher salt

Directions:

1. Supply your smoker with wood pellets and follow the start-up procedure. Preheat the grill, with the lid closed, to 350° F.

2. Toss all ingredients together and spread out evenly on a sheet tray.

3. Place the tray directly on the grill grate and roast until the bacon is crispy and beans are lightly browned, about 20 minutes. Enjoy! Grill: 450 ℉

Smoked & Loaded Baked Potato

Servings: 4

Cooking Time: 60 Minutes

Ingredients:

➢ 6 Yukon Gold or russet potatoes

➢ 8 Slices bacon

➢ 1/2 Cup butter, melted

➢ 1 Cup sour cream

➢ 1 1/2 Cup shredded cheddar cheese, divided

➢ salt and pepper

➢ 1 Bunch green onions, thinly sliced

Directions:

1. Supply your smoker with wood pellets and follow the start-up procedure. Preheat the grill, with the lid closed, to 375° F.

2. Poke potatoes with a fork, then place straight onto the grill. Cook for 1 hour. Grill: 375 °F

3. At the same time, cook bacon on a baking sheet on the grill for about 20 minutes; remove, cool and crumble. Grill: 375 °F

4. Once potatoes are done, remove and allow to cool for 15 minutes.

5. Cut each potato lengthwise, creating long halves. Use a small spoon to scoop out about 70% of the potato to make a boat, keeping a thick layer of potato near skin.

6. Place excess potato in a bowl and reserve. Lightly mash extra potato with a fork; add butter, sour cream, 1/2 cup cheese and season with salt and pepper.

7. Take the potato skins and fill with potato mixture, then sprinkle with extra cheese and bacon.

8. Place back on grill for about 10 minutes or until warm and cheese has melted. Garnish with green onions and extra sour cream. Enjoy! Grill: 375 °F

Grilled Chili-lime Corn

Servings: 8

Cooking Time: 45 Minutes

Ingredients:

➢ 12 Corn, ears

➢ 1 Teaspoon chili powder

➢ 1/2 Teaspoon onion powder

➢ 1 Teaspoon Leinenkugel's Summer Shandy Rub

➢ 2 lime, juiced

➢ 1 Tablespoon lime zest

Directions:

1. Soak the ears of corn, still in their husk, in water for 4 to 8 hours.

2. Supply your smoker with wood pellets and follow the start-up procedure. Preheat the grill, with the lid closed, to 350° F.

3. Place corn directly on grill grates. Turn corn every 15 minutes for 45 minutes total cooking time. Grill: 350 °F

4. Combine chili powder, onion powder, Summer Shandy rub, lime juice, lime zest and butter in an oven safe dish and place in grill for 10 minutes. Remove corn and butter from the grill.

5. Pull corn husk back, but not off and remove corn silk. Using the corn husk as a handle, brush the corn with the melted chili-lime butter. Enjoy!

Roasted Red Pepper White Bean Dip

Servings: 4   Cooking Time: 40 Minutes

Ingredients:

- 4 Whole garlic
- 4 Tablespoon extra-virgin olive oil
- 2 Bell Pepper, Red
- 3 Tablespoon Dill Weed, fresh

- 3 Tablespoon chopped flat-leaf parsley
- 2 Can cannellini beans, mashed
- 4 Teaspoon lemon juice
- 1 1/2 Teaspoon salt

Directions:

1. Roasting the garlic and red peppers:

2. Supply your smoker with wood pellets and follow the start-up procedure. Preheat the grill, with the lid closed, to 400° F.

3. Peel away the outside layers of the garlic husk. Cut off the top of the garlic bulb, exposing each of the individual cloves. Drizzle olive oil over the top of the head of garlic and rub it in. Wrap the garlic in foil, completely covering it. Put the head of garlic and the two red peppers (washed and dried) on the Traeger.

4. Roast the garlic for 25-30 minutes and the peppers for about 40 minutes. Rotate the peppers a quarter-turn every 10 minutes until the exterior is blistered and blackened. Grill: 400 °F

5. Pull the peppers off the grill and put them in a bowl. Cover the bowl with plastic wrap and leave them for 15 minutes. The steam will loosen the skins so that they slip off like a drumstick covered in barbecue sauce.

6. Peel off the pepper skin. Cut off the stems and scrape out the seeds and they're ready to use.

7. As for the garlic, let it cool and then pull out the individual cloves as needed.

8. The dip:

9. In a blender put the roasted red peppers, 4 cloves of roasted garlic, dill, parsley, drained and rinsed beans, olive oil, lemon juice and salt.

10. Blend until the dip is smooth and creamy. You may need to scrape down the sides of the blender a couple of times. If it's having difficulty blending or looks too thick add more olive oil or lemon juice. (Add more lemon juice if it tastes like it needs more acid or brightness.) Enjoy!

Tater Tot Bake

Servings: 4

Cooking Time: 15 Minutes

Ingredients:

- ➤ 1 Whole frozen tater tots
- ➤ salt and pepper
- ➤ 1 Cup sour cream
- ➤ 1 Cup shredded cheddar cheese, divided
- ➤ 1/2 Cup bacon, chopped
- ➤ 1/4 Cup green onion, diced

Directions:

1. Supply your smoker with wood pellets and follow the start-up procedure. Preheat the grill, with the lid closed, to 375° F.

2. Line a baking sheet with aluminum foil for easy clean up and spread frozen tater tots onto sheet.

3. Sprinkle with Veggie Shake or salt and pepper to taste.

4. Place the baking sheet on the preheated grill grate and cook the tater tots for 10 minutes.

5. Drizzle sour cream over cooked tater tots.

6. Sprinkle the cheese, bacon bits and green onions on top of the tater tots.

7. Turn heat up to High heat and cook for 5 more minutes until the cheese melts and serve immediately. Enjoy!

Roasted Sweet Potato Steak Fries

Servings: 4

Cooking Time: 40 Minutes

Ingredients:

➤ 3 Whole sweet potatoes

➤ 4 Tablespoon extra-virgin olive oil

➤ salt and pepper

➤ 2 Tablespoon fresh chopped rosemary

Directions:

1. Supply your smoker with wood pellets and follow the start-up procedure. Preheat the grill, with the lid closed, to 450° F.

2. Cut sweet potatoes into wedges and toss with olive oil, salt, pepper and rosemary. Spread on a parchment lined baking sheet and put in the grill. Cook for 15 minutes then flip and continue to cook until lightly browned and cooked through, about 40 to 45 minutes total. Grill: 450 °F

3. Serve with your favorite dipping sauce. Enjoy! Grill: 450 °F

Roasted Potato Poutine

Servings: 6

Cooking Time: 40 Minutes

Ingredients:

➢ 4 Large russet potatoes

➢ Tablespoon olive oil or vegetable oil

➢ Prime Rib Rub

➢ Cup chicken or beef gravy (homemade or jarred)

➢ 1 1/2 Cup white or yellow cheddar cheese curds

➢ freshly ground black pepper

➢ 2 Tablespoon scallions

Directions:

1. Supply your smoker with wood pellets and follow the start-up procedure. Preheat the grill, with the lid closed, to 500° F.

2. Scrub the potatoes and slice into fries, wedges or preferred shape.

3. Put potatoes into a large mixing bowl and coat with oil. Season generously with Traeger Prime Rib rub.

4. Tip the potatoes onto a rimmed baking sheet and spread in a single layer, cut sides down.

5. Roast for 20 minutes, then using a spatula, turn the potatoes to the other cut side. Continue to roast until the potatoes are tender and golden brown, about 15 to 20 minutes more.

6. While potatoes cook, warm the gravy on the stovetop or in a heat-proof saucepan on your Traeger.

7. To assemble the poutine, arrange the potatoes in a large shallow bowl or on a serving platter. Distribute the cheese curds on top. Pour the hot gravy evenly over the potatoes and cheese curds.

8. Season with black pepper and garnish with thinly sliced scallions. Serve immediately. Enjoy!

Smoked Mushrooms

Servings: 4

Cooking Time: 45 Minutes

Ingredients:

➤ Pound Mushrooms, fresh

➤ 1/2 Cup apple cider vinegar

➤ 1/2 Cup soy sauce

➤ 1 Teaspoon Blackened Saskatchewan Rub

Directions:

1. Clean mushrooms and place in a large Ziploc bag. Add apple cider vinegar, soy sauce and rub.

2. Mix well and allow to marinate in the refrigerator for at least 2 hours.

3. Supply your smoker with wood pellets and follow the start-up procedure. Preheat the grill, with the lid closed, to 350° F.

4. Place cast iron skillet inside grill for 20 minutes to warm up.

5. Add the mushrooms and marinade slowly into the cast iron skillet.

6. Cook uncovered for 15 minutes, then cover the skillet and cook another 30 minutes until mushrooms are tender. Grill: 350 ˚F

7. Remove skillet from grill and let mushrooms cool down for 5 minutes before serving. Enjoy!

BEEF LAMB AND GAME RECIPES

Spatchcocked Quail With Smoked Fruit

Servings: 4

Cooking Time: 60 Minutes

Ingredients:

➢ 4 quail, spatchcocked

➢ 2 teaspoons salt

➢ 2 teaspoons freshly ground black pepper

➢ 2 teaspoons garlic powder

➢ 4 ripe peaches or pears

➢ 4 tablespoons (½ stick) salted butter, softened

➢ 1 tablespoon sugar

➢ 1 teaspoon ground cinnamon

Directions:

1. Supply your smoker with wood pellets and follow the start-up procedure. Preheat, with the lid closed, to 225°F.

2. Season the quail all over with the salt, pepper, and garlic powder.

3. Cut the peaches (or pears) in half and remove the pits (or the cores).

4. In a small bowl, combine the butter, sugar, and cinnamon; set aside.

5. Arrange the quail on the grill grate, close the lid, and smoke for about 1 hour, or until a meat thermometer inserted in the thickest part reads 145°F.

6. After the quail has been cooking for about 15 minutes, add the peaches (or pears) to the grill, flesh-side down, and smoke for 30 to 40 minutes.

7. Top the cooked peaches (or pears) with the cinnamon butter and serve alongside the quail.

Smoked Longhorn Cowboy Tri-tip

Servings: 6

Cooking Time: 240 Minutes

Ingredients:

➢ 1 (2-3 lb) tri-tip

➢ 1/8 Cup coffee grounds

➢ 1/4 Cup Beef Rub

Directions:

1. Supply your smoker with wood pellets and follow the start-up procedure. Preheat the grill, with the lid closed, to 180° F.

2. Rub tri-tip with Traeger Beef Rub and coffee grounds. Place on the grill grate and smoke at 180°F for 3 hours. Grill: 180 °F

3. Remove tri-tip and increase the grill temperature to 275°F. Grill: 275 °F

4. Double wrap the tri-tip in foil, return to grill and let cook for 45 to 90 minutes, or until the internal temperature reaches 130°F to 135°F. Grill: 275 °F Probe: 135 °F

5. Remove from the grill, unwrap foil and let it rest for 10 minutes before slicing. Enjoy!

Steak Tips With Mashed Potatoes

Servings: 4-6

Cooking Time: 60 Minutes

Ingredients:

- ➢ 1 Cup Beef Broth
- ➢ 1 Stick (Room Temperature) Butter, Unsalted
- ➢ 2 Tablespoon Flour, All-Purpose
- ➢ 1 Tablespoon Java Chophouse Seasoning
- ➢ 4 Tablespoon Java Chophouse Seasoning, Divided
- ➢ 2 Pounds Medium Russet Potatoes, Peeled And Cut (Large Chunks)
- ➢ 2 Pounds Strip Sirloin
- ➢ 1/2 To 1 Cup Whole Milk, Warm

Directions:

1. For the mashed potatoes: add the potatoes to a large pot and add enough cold water to cover the potatoes. Bring to a simmer over medium heat until the potatoes are tender enough to be pierced with a fork, about 40 minutes. Drain the potatoes.

2. Add the potatoes to a large mixing bowl. Add the butter, 1 tablespoon of Java Chop House and ½ cup of warm milk. Mash until smooth and lump free. If potatoes are too thick, add more milk, a tablespoon at a time, until you reach your desired consistency.

3. For the steak tips: Supply your smoker with wood pellets and follow the start-up procedure. Preheat the grill, with the lid closed, to 350° F. Season the steaks generously on both sides with 2 tablespoons of Java Chop House seasoning and grill for 8-10 minutes per side. When steaks are done, remove from grill, allow to rest for 15 minutes, then cut into chunks.

4. While the steak is resting, add the butter to a small saucepan over low heat. Once the butter is melted, whisk in the flour and cook for 2 minutes until the flour smells toasted. Slowly whisk in the beef broth and remaining 2 tablespoons of Java Chop House seasoning and cook the gravy over low heat until thickened. Remove from heat and toss the steak tips in the gravy.

5. Serve steak tips over mashed potatoes. Enjoy!

Bbq Brisket Tomato Queso

Servings: 6

Cooking Time: 15 Minutes

Ingredients:

- ½ Cup Barbecue Sauce
- 1 Cup Brisket, Pulled
- 2 Tablespoons Butter
- 1 Pound American Or Velveeta Cheese, Cubed
- 1 Cup Green Chili, Chopped
- 1 Cup Heavy Cream
- Serving Pickled Jalapeno
- Serving Salsa
- 1 Cup Tomato, Diced
- Serving Tortilla Chip
- ½ Of One Finely Diced White Onions

Directions:

1. Supply your smoker with wood pellets and follow the start-up procedure. Preheat the grill, with the lid closed, to 300° F. If you're using gas or charcoal, set your grill for medium low, indirect heat.

2. Let the grilling skillet heat up on the grill. Then, add the 2 tablespoons of butter and finely diced onion and sauté the onions until they are soft and translucent.

3. Next, pour in the heavy cream and bring it to a simmer. Once the cream is simmering, add the cubed cheese, diced tomatoes, and chopped green chilis. Make sure to stir the mixture consistently until the cheese is completely melted.

4. In a separate bowl, combine the brisket with the barbecue sauce and toss until the brisket is fully covered.

5. When your queso is ready, pour it into a serving bowl and top with the brisket, salsa, and jalapenos. You can even add fresh cilantro as a garnish.

6. Serve the queso with tortilla chips while it's hot and fresh and enjoy.

Easy Tri Tip Shepherd's Pie

Servings: 4

Cooking Time: 30 Minutes

Ingredients:

➢ 1 Cup Beef Broth

➢ 2 Tablespoons Unsalted Butter

➢ 2 Tablespoons Chophouse Steak Seasoning

➢ 2 Tablespoons Flour

➢ 1 Cup Mashed Potatoes, Prepared

➢ 2 Cups Tri-Tip, Diced

➢ 2 Cups Mixed Frozen Vegetables, Thawed

Directions:

1. Supply your smoker with wood pellets and follow the start-up procedure. Preheat the grill, with the lid closed, to 350° F.

2. In the sauce pan, add the butter and flour over medium low heat. Cook the flour and butter for about 1 minute, or until the flour smells toasty. Slowly add in the beef broth, whisking constantly. Cook for 5 minutes, or until the gravy is thick, and then add the Chophouse Steak. Set aside.

3. Toss the vegetables and tri-tip with the gravy and divide equally into the ramekins. Top the ramekins with mashed potatoes and grill the shepherd's pies for 10-15 minutes, or until warm all the way through and the filling is bubbling. Remove from the grill and serve immediately.

Smoked New York Steaks

Servings: 4

Cooking Time: 120 Minutes

Ingredients:

- ➢ 4 (1-inch-thick) New York steaks
- ➢ 2 tablespoons olive oil
- ➢ Salt
- ➢ Freshly ground black pepper

Directions:

1. Supply your smoker with wood pellets and follow the start-up procedure. Preheat the grill, with the lid closed, to 180°F.

2. Rub the steaks all over with olive oil and season both sides with salt and pepper.

3. Place the steaks directly on the grill grate and smoke for 1 hour.

4. Increase the grill's temperature to 375°F and continue to cook until the steaks' internal temperature reaches 145°F for medium-rare.

5. Remove the steaks and let them rest 5 minutes, before slicing and serving.

Italian Meatballs

Servings: 6

Cooking Time: 90 Minutes

Ingredients:

- 1lb (450g) ground beef (85/15), well chilled
- ½lb (225g) Italian sausage, well chilled
- 1 large egg, beaten
- ½ cup finely grated Parmesan, Asiago, or Romano cheese
- ½ cup panko or other breadcrumbs
- 1 tsp Italian seasoning
- 1 tsp coarse salt
- ½ tsp freshly ground black pepper
- 1lb (450g) thin-sliced bacon, halved crosswise
- low-carb barbecue sauce, (optional)

Directions:

1. Supply your smoker with wood pellets and follow the start-up procedure. Preheat the grill, with the lid closed, to 250° F.

2. Place the ground beef, Italian sausage, egg, cheese, breadcrumbs, Italian seasoning, and salt and pepper in a large bowl. Wet your hands with cold water. Form your hands into claw shapes and combine the ingredients using a light touch.

3. Form the mixture into 24 equal-sized balls. Wrap each with a half strip of bacon and secure the ends with a toothpick.

4. Place the meatballs on the grate and smoke until the bacon has rendered its fat and the internal temperature reaches 160°F (71°C), about 1 to 1½ hours. Brush the meatballs with barbecue sauce (if using) during the last 10 minutes of smoking.

5. Transfer the meatballs to a platter. Let rest for 5 minutes before serving.

Bison Meatballs

Servings: 8 - 10   Cooking Time: 30 Minutes

Ingredients:

- 1 Cored, Peeled, And Chopped Apple
- 2 Tablespoons Beef & Brisket Rub
- 2 Cups Beef Broth
- 2 Pounds Ground Bison
- ¼ Cup Breadcrumbs
- 3 Tablespoons Cornstarch
- 2 Tablespoons Dijon Mustard
- 2 Beaten Eggs

- 1 Finely Garlic Clove, Minced
- 2 Cups Hard Cider
- 3 Tablespoons Pure Maple Syrup
- 2 Tablespoons Olive Oil
- ½ Cup Pureed Onion
- ¼ Pound Pancetta
- 3 Tablespoons Water
- 1 Thinly Sliced Yellow Onion

Directions:

1. First, make the mustard sauce. In a large saucepan, add the olive oil over medium heat, then add the onion and apple. Cook the apple and onion until soft and caramelized, about 10-12 minutes. Once the onion and apple are soft, add in the hard cider, beef broth, maple syrup and Dijon mustard to the pan. Whisk everything together and bring the sauce to a boil.

2. Once the sauce comes to a boil, reduce it to a simmer and cook, stirring and scraping the bottom of the pot occasionally until the sauce reduces by half, about 30 minutes. Remove the sauce from the heat and allow it to cool.

3. Pour the sauce into a blender, place the lid on top, and blend the sauce until completely smooth. Return the sauce into the saucepan and bring it back to a boil. In a small bowl, mix together the cornstarch and water, then pour into the sauce. Cook the sauce until thickened, whisking the entire time, about 2 minutes. Set the sauce aside.

4. Make the meatballs. In a food processor, blend the pancetta until it becomes a smooth paste. Scrape the pancetta into large mixing bowl, and mix it with the ground bison, pureed onion, eggs, breadcrumbs, garlic, and Beef and Brisket Rub. Gently mix the meat together and, using a cookie scoop, scoop into meatballs. Place the meatballs on a baking sheet. Repeat with the remaining meat mixture.

5. Supply your smoker with wood pellets and follow the start-up procedure. Preheat the grill, with the lid closed, to 350° F. If you're using a gas or charcoal grill, set it up for medium heat. Place a large cast iron skillet on the grill and add the olive oil to it. Place the meatballs in an even layer in the skillet and grill, turning the meatballs occasionally until they are browned on all sides. Insert a temperature probe into one of the meatballs and continue grilling them until the internal temperature reaches 160°F.

6. Remove the meatballs from the grill, toss them with the mustard sauce, and serve immediately.

Smoked Beef Back Ribs

Servings: 6

Cooking Time: 480 Minutes

Ingredients:

- ➤ 2 Rack beef back ribs
- ➤ 1/2 Cup Beef Rub

Directions:

1. If your butcher has not already done so, remove the thin papery membrane from the bone-side of the ribs by working the tip of a butter knife underneath the membrane over a middle bone. Use paper towels to get a firm grip, then tear the membrane off.

2. Season both sides of ribs with Traeger Beef Rub.

3. Supply your smoker with wood pellets and follow the start-up procedure. Preheat the grill, with the lid closed, to 225° F.

4. Arrange the ribs on the grill grate, bone side down. Cook for 8-10 hours, or until internal temperature reaches 205°F. Grill: 225 °F Probe: 205 °F

5. Remove ribs from grill and let rest, lightly covered for 20 minutes before slicing and serving. Enjoy!

Grilled Loco Moco Burger

Servings: 4

Cooking Time: 10 Minutes

Ingredients:

➢ Ounce ground beef, 80% lean

➢ 3 Tablespoon kosher salt

➢ 2 Tablespoon black pepper

➢ Cup Beef Gravy

➢ 2 Cup Rice, Cooked

➢ 4 eggs

➢ burger buns

➢ 2 Cup Hawaiian Pasta Salad

Directions:

1. Supply your smoker with wood pellets and follow the start-up procedure. Preheat the grill, with the lid closed, to 375° F.

2. Divide the ground beef into four, 6 oz portions and shape into patties. Season the patties with salt and pepper.

3. Place the patties on the grill and flip after six minutes cook time.

4. Check the internal temperature of the patties. Burgers are done when they reach an internal temperature of 165°F. Probe: 165 °F

5. While the patties are cooking, heat the gravy and the rice. Cook the eggs over easy.

6. To assemble the burger: Start with the bottom of the bun, 1/4 cup rice, 1/4 cup pasta salad, a hamburger patty, gravy, a fried egg, and the top of the bun.

7. Serve while hot. Enjoy!

Bbq Burnt End Sandwich

Servings: 2

Cooking Time: 480 Minutes

Ingredients:

- ➢ 1 point cut brisket
- ➢ Beef Rub
- ➢ 1/2 Cup beef broth
- ➢ 1 Cup Texas Spicy BBQ Sauce
- ➢ 4 Slices Monterey Jack cheese
- ➢ 4 burger buns

Directions:

1. Supply your smoker with wood pellets and follow the start-up procedure. Preheat the grill, with the lid closed, to 250° F.

2. Trim excess fat off brisket point. Season brisket point liberally with Traeger Beef rub.

3. Place brisket point directly on the grill grate. Cook until it reaches an internal temperature of 170℉, approximately 4 to 5 hours. Grill: 250 ℉

4. Remove brisket from grill and cut into 1-inch cubes. Add the beef broth to the pan with the cubed brisket. Cover pan with aluminum foil.

5. Place pan in grill and cook for 90 minutes. Grill: 250 ℉

6. Remove the foil and add Traeger Texas Spicy BBQ sauce. Stir and put back on the grill, uncovered, for an additional 45 minutes. Remove from grill. Grill: 250 ℉

7. Top each bun with the burnt ends, cheese, and additional BBQ sauce. Enjoy!

APPETIZERS AND SNACKS

Grilled Guacamole

Servings: 6

Cooking Time: 30 Minutes

Ingredients:

- 3 large avocados, halved and pitted
- 1 lime, halved
- ½ jalapeño, deseeded and deveined
- ½ small white or red onion, peeled
- 2 garlic cloves, peeled and skewered on a toothpick
- 1 tsp coarse salt, plus more
- 1½ tbsp reduced-fat mayo
- 2 tbsp chopped fresh cilantro
- 2 tbsp crumbled queso fresco (optional)
- tortilla chips

Directions:

1. Supply your smoker with wood pellets and follow the start-up procedure. Preheat the grill, with the lid closed, to 225° F.

2. Place the avocados, lime, jalapeño, and onion cut sides down on the grate. Use the toothpicks to balance the garlic cloves between the bars. Smoke for 30 minutes. (You want the vegetables to retain most of their rawness.)

3. Transfer everything to a cutting board. Remove the garlic cloves from the toothpick and roughly chop. Sprinkle with the salt and continue to mince the garlic until it begins to form a paste. Scrape the garlic and salt into a large bowl.

4. Scoop the avocado flesh from the peels into the bowl. Squeeze the juice of ½ lime over the avocado. Mash the avocados but leave them somewhat chunky. Finely dice the jalapeño. Dice 2 tablespoons of onion. (Reserve the remaining onion for another use.) Add the jalapeño, onion, mayo, and cilantro to the bowl. Stir gently to combine. Taste for seasoning, adding more salt, lime juice, and jalapeño as desired.

5. Transfer the guacamole to a serving bowl. Top with the queso fresco (if using). Serve with tortilla chips.

Delicious Deviled Crab Appetizer

Servings: 30

Cooking Time: 10 Minutes

Ingredients:

- Nonstick cooking spray, oil, or butter, for greasing
- 1 cup panko breadcrumbs, divided
- 1 cup canned corn, drained
- ½ cup chopped scallions, divided
- ½ red bell pepper, finely chopped
- 16 ounces jumbo lump crabmeat
- ¾ cup mayonnaise, divided
- 1 egg, beaten
- 1 teaspoon salt
- 1 teaspoon freshly ground black pepper
- 2 teaspoons cayenne pepper, divided
- Juice of 1 lemon

Directions:

1. Supply your smoker with wood pellets and follow the start-up procedure. Preheat, with the lid closed, to 425°F.

2. Spray three 12-cup mini muffin pans with cooking spray and divide ½ cup of the panko between 30 of the muffin cups, pressing into the bottoms and up the sides. (Work in batches, if necessary, depending on the number of pans you have.)

3. In a medium bowl, combine the corn, ¼ cup of scallions, the bell pepper, crabmeat, half of the mayonnaise, the egg, salt, pepper, and 1 teaspoon of cayenne pepper.

4. Gently fold in the remaining ½ cup of breadcrumbs and divide the mixture between the prepared mini muffin cups.

5. Place the pans on the grill grate, close the lid, and smoke for 10 minutes, or until golden brown.

6. In a small bowl, combine the lemon juice and the remaining mayonnaise, scallions, and cayenne pepper to make a sauce.

7. Brush the tops of the mini crab cakes with the sauce and serve hot.

Smoked Cashews

Servings: 6

Cooking Time: 60 Minutes

Ingredients:

➢ 1 pound roasted, salted cashews

Directions:

1. Supply your smoker with wood pellets and follow the start-up procedure. Preheat the grill, with the lid closed, to 120°F.

2. Pour the cashews onto a rimmed baking sheet and smoke for 1 hour, stirring once about halfway through the smoking time.

3. Remove the cashews from the grill, let cool, and store in an airtight container for as long as you can resist.

Pulled Pork Loaded Nachos

Servings: 4   Cooking Time: 10 Minutes

Ingredients:

- 2 cups leftover smoked pulled pork
- 1 small sweet onion, diced
- 1 medium tomato, diced
- 1 jalapeño pepper, seeded and diced
- 1 garlic clove, minced
- 1 teaspoon salt
- 1 teaspoon freshly ground black pepper
- 1 bag tortilla chips

- 1 cup shredded Cheddar cheese
- ½ cup The Ultimate BBQ Sauce, divided
- ½ cup shredded jalapeño Monterey Jack cheese
- Juice of ½ lime
- 1 avocado, halved, pitted, and sliced
- 2 tablespoons sour cream
- 1 tablespoon chopped fresh cilantro

Directions:

1. Supply your smoker with wood pellets and follow the start-up procedure. Preheat, with the lid closed, to 375°F.

2. Heat the pulled pork in the microwave.

3. In a medium bowl, combine the onion, tomato, jalapeño, garlic, salt, and pepper, and set aside.

4. Arrange half of the tortilla chips in a large cast iron skillet. Spread half of the warmed pork on top and cover with the Cheddar cheese. Top with half of the onion-jalapeño mixture, then drizzle with ¼ cup of barbecue sauce.

5. Layer on the remaining tortilla chips, then the remaining pork and the Monterey Jack cheese. Top with the remaining onion-jalapeño mixture and drizzle with the remaining ¼ cup of barbecue sauce.

6. Place the skillet on the grill, close the lid, and smoke for about 10 minutes, or until the cheese is melted and bubbly. (Watch to make sure your chips don't burn!)

7. Squeeze the lime juice over the nachos, top with the avocado slices and sour cream, and garnish with the cilantro before serving hot.

Chuckwagon Beef Jerky

Servings: 6   Cooking Time: 300 Minutes

Ingredients:

- 2½lb (1.2kg) boneless top or bottom round steak, sirloin tip, flank steak, or venison
- 1 cup sugar-free dark-colored soda
- 1 cup cold brewed coffee
- ½ cup light soy sauce
- ¼ cup Worcestershire sauce
- 2 tbsp whiskey (optional)
- 2 tsp chili powder
- 1½ tsp garlic salt
- 1 tsp onion powder
- 1 tsp pink curing salt

Directions:

1. Slice the meat into ¼-inch-thick (.5cm) strips, trimming off any visible fat or gristle. (Slice against the grain for more tender jerky and with the grain for chewier jerky.) Place the meat in a large resealable plastic bag.

2. In a small bowl, whisk together the soda, coffee, soy sauce, Worcestershire sauce, whiskey (if using), chili powder, garlic salt, onion powder, and curing salt (if using). Whisk until the salt dissolves. Pour the mixture over the meat and reseal the bag. Refrigerate for 24 to 48 hours, turning the bag several times to redistribute the brine.

3. Supply your smoker with wood pellets and follow the start-up procedure. Preheat the grill, with the lid closed, to 150° F.

4. Drain the meat and discard the brine. Place the strips of meat in a single layer on paper towels and blot any excess moisture.

5. Place the meat in a single layer on the grate and smoke for 4 to 5 hours, turning once or twice. (If you're aware of hot spots on your grate, rotate the strips so they smoke evenly.) To test for doneness, bend one or two pieces in the middle. They should be dry but still somewhat pliant. Or simply eat a piece to see if it's done to your liking.

6. For the best texture, when you remove the meat from the grill, place the still-warm jerky in a resealable plastic bag and let rest for 30 minutes. (You might see condensation form on the inside of the bag, but the moisture will be reabsorbed by the meat.) Or let the meat cool completely and then store in a resealable plastic bag or covered container. The jerky will last a few days at room temperature but will last longer (up to 2 weeks) if refrigerated.

Sriracha & Maple Cashews

Servings: 10

Cooking Time: 60 Minutes

Ingredients:

➢ 2 tbsp unsalted butter

➢ 3 tbsp pure maple syrup

➢ 1 tbsp sriracha

➢ 1 tsp coarse salt (use only if nuts are unsalted)

➢ 2½ cups unsalted cashews

Directions:

1. Supply your smoker with wood pellets and follow the start-up procedure. Preheat the grill, with the lid closed, to 250° F.

2. In a small saucepan on the stovetop over low heat, melt the butter. Add the maple syrup, sriracha, and salt (if using). Stir until combined. Add the nuts and stir gently to coat thoroughly.

3. Spread the nuts in a single layer in an aluminum foil roasting pan coated with cooking spray. Place the pan on the grate and smoke the nuts until they're lightly toasted, about 1 hour, stirring once or twice.

4. Remove the pan from the grill and let the nuts cool for 15 minutes. They'll be sticky at first but will crisp up. Break them up with your fingers and store at room temperature in an airtight container, such as a lidded glass jar.

Smoked Turkey Sandwich

Servings: 1

Cooking Time: 15 Minutes

Ingredients:

- ➢ 2 slices sourdough bread
- ➢ 2 tablespoons butter, at room temperature
- ➢ 2 (1-ounce) slices Swiss cheese
- ➢ 4 ounces leftover Smoked Turkey
- ➢ 1 teaspoon garlic salt

Directions:

1. Supply your smoker with wood pellets and follow the start-up procedure. Preheat the grill, with the lid closed, to 375°F.

2. Coat one side of each bread slice with 1 tablespoon of butter and sprinkle the buttered sides with garlic salt.

3. Place 1 slice of cheese on each unbuttered side of the bread, and then put the turkey on the cheese.

4. Close the sandwich, buttered sides out, and place it directly on the grill grate. Cook for 5 minutes. Flip the sandwich and cook for 5 minutes more. Remove the sandwich from the grill, cut it in half, and serve.

Pigs In A Blanket

Servings: 4-6

Cooking Time: 15 Minutes

Ingredients:

- ➢ 2 Tablespoon Poppy Seeds
- ➢ 1 Tablespoon Dried Minced Onion
- ➢ 2 Teaspoon garlic, minced
- ➢ 2 Tablespoon Sesame Seeds
- ➢ 1 Teaspoon salt
- ➢ 8 Ounce Original Crescent Dough
- ➢ 1/4 Cup Dijon mustard
- ➢ 1 Large egg, beaten

Directions:

1. When ready to cook, start your smoker at 350 degrees F, and preheat with lid closed, 10 to 15 minutes.

2. Mix together poppy seeds, dried minced onion, dried minced garlic, salt and sesame seeds. Set aside.

3. Cut each triangle of crescent roll dough into thirds lengthwise, making 3 small strips from each roll.

4. Brush the dough strips lightly with Dijon mustard. Put the mini hot dogs on 1 end of the dough and roll up.

5. Arrange them, seam side down, on a greased baking pan. Brush with egg wash and sprinkle with seasoning mixture.

6. Bake in smoker until golden brown, about 12 to 15 minutes.

7. Serve with mustard or dipping sauce of your choice. Enjoy!

Bacon Pork Pinwheels (kansas Lollipops)

Servings: 4-6

Cooking Time: 20 Minutes

Ingredients:

➢ 1 Whole Pork Loin, boneless
➢ To Taste salt and pepper
➢ To Taste Greek Seasoning
➢ 4 Slices bacon
➢ To Taste The Ultimate BBQ Sauce

Directions:

1. When ready to cook, start the smoker and set temperature to 500F. Preheat, lid closed, for 10 to 15 minutes.

2. Trim pork loin of any unwanted silver skin or fat. Using a sharp knife, cut pork loin length wise, into 4 long strips.

3. Lay pork flat, then season with salt, pepper and Cavender's Greek Seasoning.

4. Flip the pork strips over and layer bacon on unseasoned side. Begin tightly rolling the pork strips, with bacon being rolled up on the inside.

5. Secure a skewer all the way through each pork roll to secure it in place. Set the pork rolls down on grill and cook for 15 minutes.

6. Brush BBQ Sauce over the pork. Turn each skewer over, then coat the other side. Let pork cook for another 5-10 minutes, depending on thickness of your pork. Enjoy!

Deviled Eggs With Smoked Paprika

Servings: 6   Cooking Time: 30 Minutes

Ingredients:

- 6 large eggs
- 3 tbsp reduced-fat mayo, plus more
- 1 tsp Dijon or yellow mustard
- ½ tsp Spanish smoked paprika or regular paprika, plus more
- dash of hot sauce
- coarse salt
- freshly ground black pepper
- for garnishing
- small sprigs of fresh parsley, dill, tarragon, or cilantro
- chopped chives
- minced scallions

- Mustard Caviar
- sliced green or black olives
- celery leaves
- sliced radishes
- diced bell peppers
- sliced cherry tomatoes
- fresh or pickled jalapeños
- sliced or diced pickles
- slivers of sun-dried tomatoes
- bacon crumbles
- smoked salmon
- Hawaiian black salt
- Caviar

Directions:

1. Supply your smoker with wood pellets and follow the start-up procedure. Preheat the grill, with the lid closed, to 180° F.

2. On the stovetop over medium-high heat, bring a saucepan of water to a boil. (Make sure there's enough water in the saucepan to cover the eggs by 1 inch [5cm].) Use a slotted spoon to gently lower the eggs into the water. Lower the heat to maintain a simmer. Set a timer for 13 minutes.

3. Prepare an ice bath by combining ice and cold water in a large bowl. Carefully transfer the eggs to the ice bath when the timer goes off.

4. When the eggs are cool enough to handle, gently tap them all over to crack the shell. Carefully peel the eggs. Rinse under cold running water to remove any clinging bits of shell, but don't dry the eggs. (A damp surface will help the smoke adhere to the egg whites.)

5. Place the eggs on the grate and smoke until the eggs take on a light brown patina from the smoke, about 25 minutes. Transfer the eggs to a cutting board, handling them as little as possible.

6. Slice each egg in half lengthwise with a sharp knife. Wipe any yolk off the blade before slicing the next egg. Gently remove the yolks and place them in a food processor. Pulse to break up the yolks. Add the mayo, mustard, paprika, and hot sauce. Season with salt and pepper to taste. Pulse until the filling is smooth. Add additional mayo 1 teaspoon at a time if the mixture is a little dry. (It shouldn't be too loose either.)

7. Spoon the filling into each egg half or pipe it in using a small resealable plastic bag. You can also use a pastry bag fitted with a fluted tip.

8. Place the eggs on a platter and lightly dust with paprika. Accompany with one or more of the suggested garnishes.

Chicken Wings With Teriyaki Glaze

Servings: 4   Cooking Time: 50 Minutes

Ingredients:

- 16 large chicken wings, about 3lb (1.4kg) total
- 1 to 1½ tbsp toasted sesame oil
- for the glaze
- ½ cup light soy sauce or tamari
- ¼ cup sake or sugar-free dark-colored soda
- ¼ cup light brown sugar or low-carb substitute
- 2 tbsp mirin or 1 tbsp honey

- 1 garlic clove, peeled, minced or grated
- 2 tsp minced fresh ginger
- 1 tsp cornstarch mixed with 1 tbsp distilled water (optional)
- for serving
- 1 tbsp toasted sesame seeds
- 2 scallions, trimmed, white and green parts sliced sharply diagonally

Directions:

1. Supply your smoker with wood pellets and follow the start-up procedure. Preheat the grill, with the lid closed, to 350° F.

2. Place the chicken wings in a large bowl, add the sesame oil, and turn the wings to coat thoroughly.

3. Place the wings on the grate at an angle to the bars. Grill for 20 minutes and then turn. Continue to cook until the wings are nicely browned and the meat is no longer pink at the bone, about 20 minutes more.

4. To make the glaze, in a saucepan on the stovetop over medium-high heat, combine the ingredients and bring the mixture to a boil. Reduce the glaze by 1/3, about 6 to 8 minutes. If you prefer your glaze to be glossy and thick, add the cornstarch and water mixture to the glaze and cook until it coats the back of a spoon, about 1 to 2 minutes more.

5. Transfer the wings to an aluminum foil roasting pan. Pour the glaze over them, turning to coat thoroughly. Place the pan on the grate and cook the wings until the glaze sets, about 5 to 10 minutes.

6. Transfer the wings to a platter. Scatter the sesame seeds and scallions over the top. Serve with plenty of napkins.

Bayou Wings With Cajun Rémoulade

Servings: 8   Cooking Time: 40 Minutes

Ingredients:

- 16 large whole chicken wings or 32 drumettes and flats, about 3lb (1.4kg) total
- for the rub
- 1 tbsp kosher salt
- 1 tsp freshly ground black pepper
- 1 tsp paprika
- ½ tsp ground cayenne, plus more
- ½ tsp garlic powder
- ½ tsp celery salt
- ½ tsp dried thyme
- 2 tbsp vegetable oil
- for the rémoulade

- 1¼ cups reduced-fat mayo
- ¼ cup Creole-style or whole grain mustard
- 2 tbsp horseradish
- 2 tbsp pickle relish
- 1 tbsp freshly squeezed lemon juice
- 1 tsp paprika, plus more
- 1 tsp hot sauce, plus more
- 1 tsp Worcestershire sauce
- coarse salt
- for serving
- lemon wedges
- pickled okra (optional)

Directions:

1. Supply your smoker with wood pellets and follow the start-up procedure. Preheat the grill, with the lid closed, to 350° F.

2. If using whole wings, cut through the two joints, separating them into drumettes, flats, and wing tips. (Discard the wing tips or save them for chicken stock.) Alternatively, leave the wings whole. Place the chicken in a resealable plastic bag.

3. In a small bowl, make the rub by combining the ingredients. Mix well. Pour the rub over the wings and toss them to thoroughly coat. Refrigerate for 2 hours.

4. In a small bowl, make the Cajun rémoulade by whisking together the mayo, mustard, horseradish, pickle relish, lemon juice, paprika, hot sauce, and Worcestershire. Season with salt to taste. The mixture should be highly seasoned. Transfer to a serving bowl and lightly dust with paprika. Cover and refrigerate until ready to serve.

5. Remove the wings from the refrigerator and allow the excess marinade to drip off. Place the wings on the grate at an angle to the bars. Grill for 20 minutes and then turn. (They'll brown more evenly but will also have less of a tendency to stick.) Continue to cook until the wings are nicely browned and the meat is no longer pink at the bone, about 20 minutes more.

6. Remove the wings from the grill and pile them on a platter. Serve with the Cajun rémoulade, lemon wedges, and pickled okra (if using).

COCKTAILS RECIPES

Garden Gimlet Cocktail

Servings: 2

Cooking Time: 45 Minutes

Ingredients:

➢ 2 Cup honey

➢ 4 lemons, zested

➢ 4 Sprig rosemary, plus more for garnish

➢ 1/2 Cup water

➢ 4 Slices cucumber

➢ 1 1/2 Ounce lime juice

➢ 3 Ounce vodka

Directions:

1. Supply your smoker with wood pellets and follow the start-up procedure. Preheat the grill, with the lid closed, to 180° F.

2. To make smoked lemon and rosemary honey syrup, thin 1 cup honey by adding 1/4 cup water to a shallow pan. Add lemon zest and 2 sprigs rosemary.

3. Place the pan directly on the grill grate and smoke 45 minutes to an hour. Remove from heat, strain and cool. Grill: 180 °F

4. In a cocktail shaker, muddle the cucumbers and 1oz of the smoked lemon and rosemary honey syrup.

5. After muddling, add lime juice, vodka, and ice. Shake and double strain into a coup glass.

6. Garnish with a sprig of rosemary. Enjoy!

Bacon Old-fashioned Cocktail

Servings: 2

Cooking Time: 20 Minutes

Ingredients:

- ➢ 16 Slices bacon
- ➢ 1/2 Cup warm water (110°F to 115°F)
- ➢ 1500 mL bourbon
- ➢ 1/2 Fluid Ounce maple syrup
- ➢ 4 Dash Angostura bitters
- ➢ 2 fresh orange peel

Directions:

1. Smoke bacon prior to making Old Fashioned using this recipe for Applewood Smoked Bacon.

2. To Make Bacon: Supply your smoker with wood pellets and follow the start-up procedure. Preheat the grill, with the lid closed, to 325° F.

3. Place bacon in a single layer on a cooling rack that fits inside a baking sheet pan. Cook in Traeger for 15-20 minutes or until bacon is browned and crispy. Reserve bacon for later. Let the fat cool slightly; you'll use the fat to infuse the bourbon. Grill: 325 °F

4. Combine 1/4 cup of warm (not hot) liquid bacon fat with the entire contents of a 750ml bottle of bourbon in a glass or heavy plastic container.

5. Use a fork to stir well. Let it sit on the counter for a few hours, stirring every so often.

6. After about four hours, put bourbon fat mixture into the freezer. After about an hour, the fat will congeal and you can simply scoop it out with a spoon. You can fine-strain the mixture through a sieve to remove all fat if desired.

7. Combine ingredients with ice and stir until cold. Strain over fresh ice in an Old Fashioned glass and garnish with reserved bacon and orange peel. Enjoy!

Fig Slider Cocktail

Servings: 2

Cooking Time: 15 Minutes

Ingredients:

➢ 2 peach, halved

➢ 4 oranges

➢ honey

➢ sugar

➢ 2 Teaspoon orange fig spread

➢ 1 Ounce fresh lemon juice

➢ 4 Ounce bourbon

➢ 3 Ounce honey glazed grilled orange juice

Directions:

1. Supply your smoker with wood pellets and follow the start-up procedure. Preheat the grill, with the lid closed, to 325° F.

2. Pit the peach and cut in half. Cut one of the oranges in half. Glaze the peach and orange cut sides with honey and set directly on the grill grate until the honey caramelizes and fruit has grill marks. Grill: 325 °F

3. Cut the second orange into wheels and coat with granulated sugar on both sides. Place directly on the grill grate and cook 15 minutes each side or until grill marks form. Grill: 325 °F

4. In a mixing tin, add grilled peaches, bourbon, orange fig spread, fresh lemon juice and honey glazed orange juice.

5. Shake vigorously to blend the juices and fig spread. Strain over clean ice. Garnish with grilled orange wheel. Enjoy!

Batter Up Cocktail

Servings: 2

Cooking Time: 60 Minutes

Ingredients:

- ➢ 2 whole nutmeg
- ➢ 4 Ounce Michter's Bourbon
- ➢ 3 Teaspoon pumpkin puree
- ➢ 1 Ounce Smoked Simple Syrup
- ➢ 2 Large egg

Directions:

1. Supply your smoker with wood pellets and follow the start-up procedure. Preheat the grill, with the lid closed, to 180° F.

2. Place whole nutmeg on a sheet tray and place in the grill. Smoke 1 hour. Remove from grill and let cool. Grill: 180 ℉

3. Add everything to a shaker and shake without ice. Add ice, then shake and strain into a chilled highball glass.

4. Garnish with grated, smoked nutmeg. Enjoy!

Smoked Hibiscus Sparkler

Servings: 4

Cooking Time: 30 Minutes

Ingredients:

➢ 1/2 Cup sugar

➢ 2 Tablespoon dried hibiscus flowers

➢ 1 Bottle sparkling wine

➢ crystallized ginger, for garnish

Directions:

1. Supply your smoker with wood pellets and follow the start-up procedure. Preheat the grill, with the lid closed, to 180° F.

2. Place water in a shallow baking dish and place directly on the grill grate. Smoke the water for 30 minutes or until desired smoke flavor is achieved. Grill: 180 °F

3. Pour water into a small saucepan and add sugar and hibiscus flowers. Bring to a simmer over medium heat and cook until sugar is dissolved.

4. Strain out the hibiscus flowers and transfer your simple syrup to a small container and refrigerate until chilled.

5. Pour 1/2 ounce smoked hibiscus simple syrup in the bottom of a champagne glass and top with sparkling wine.

6. Drop in a few pieces of crystallized ginger to garnish. Enjoy!

Smoked Barnburner Cocktail

Servings: 2

Cooking Time: 45 Minutes

Ingredients:

- 16 Ounce fresh raspberries
- 1/2 Cup Smoked Simple Syrup
- 1 1/2 Ounce smoked raspberry syrup
- 3 Ounce reposado tequila
- 1 Ounce lime juice
- 1 Ounce lemon juice
- 2 grilled lime wheel, for garnish

Directions:

1. Supply your smoker with wood pellets and follow the start-up procedure. Preheat the grill, with the lid closed, to 180° F.

2. For Smoked Raspberry Syrup: Place fresh raspberries on a grill mat and smoke for 30 minutes. After the raspberries have been smoked, reserve a few for garnish and place the remainder into a shallow sheet pan with Traeger Smoked Simple Syrup. Grill: 180 ˚F

3. Place sheet pan on the grill grate and smoke for 45 minutes. Remove from grill and let cool. Strain through a fine mesh sieve discarding solids. Transfer the syrup to the refrigerator until ready to use. Makes about 1/2 cup of smoked raspberry syrup. Grill: 180 ˚F

4. For cocktail: Add 3/4 ounce smoked raspberry syrup, tequila, lime juice and lemon juice with ice into a mixing glass. Shake and pour over clean ice. Garnish with smoked raspberries and a grilled lime wheel. Enjoy!

Smoked Plum And Thyme Fizz Cocktail

Servings: 2

Cooking Time: 60 Minutes

Ingredients:

- 6 fresh plums
- 4 Fluid Ounce vodka
- 1 1/2 Fluid Ounce fresh lemon juice
- 2 Ounce smoked plum and thyme simple syrup
- 4 Fluid Ounce club soda
- 2 Slices smoked plum, for garnish
- 2 Sprig fresh thyme, for garnish
- 8 Sprig thyme
- 2 Cup Smoked Simple Syrup

Directions:

1. Supply your smoker with wood pellets and follow the start-up procedure. Preheat the grill, with the lid closed, to 180° F.

2. Cut plums in half and remove the pit. Place the plum halves directly on the grill grate and smoke for 25 minutes. Grill: 180 ˚F

3. For the Plum and Thyme Simple Syrup: After 25 minutes, remove plums from the grill and cut into quarters. Add plums and thyme sprigs to 1 cup of Traeger Smoked Simple Syrup. Smoke the mixture for 45 minutes. Remove from grill, strain and let cool. Grill: 180 ˚F

4. Add vodka, fresh lemon juice and smoked plum and thyme simple syrup to a mixing glass.

5. Add ice and shake. Strain over clean ice, top off with club soda and garnish with a piece of thyme and slice of smoked plum. Enjoy!

Grilled Peach Smash Cocktail

Servings: 2

Cooking Time: 10 Minutes

Ingredients:

- ➢ 2 peach, sliced and grilled
- ➢ 10 fresh mint leaves
- ➢ 1 1/2 Ounce Smoked Simple Syrup
- ➢ 4 Ounce bourbon
- ➢ 2 mint sprig, for garnish

Directions:

1. Supply your smoker with wood pellets and follow the start-up procedure. Preheat the grill, with the lid closed, to 375° F.

2. Cut the peach into 6 slices and brush with Traeger Smoked Simple Syrup. Place directly on the grill grate and cook 10 to 12 minutes or until peaches soften and get grill marks. Grill: 375 °F

3. In a mixing glass, add 3 slices of grilled peaches, 5 mint leaves and Traeger Smoked Simple Syrup.

4. Muddle ingredients to release oils of the mint and juices from the grilled peaches. Add bourbon and crushed ice.

5. Shake and pour into a stemless wine glass. Top off with more crushed ice. Garnish with a grilled peach and mint sprig. Enjoy!

Smoked Hot Buttered Rum

Servings: 4

Cooking Time: 30 Minutes

Ingredients:

- ➢ 2 Cup water
- ➢ 1/4 Cup brown sugar
- ➢ 1/2 Stick butter, melted
- ➢ 1 Teaspoon ground cinnamon
- ➢ 1/4 Teaspoon ground nutmeg
- ➢ ground cloves
- ➢ salt
- ➢ 6 Ounce Rum

Directions:

1. Supply your smoker with wood pellets and follow the start-up procedure. Preheat the grill, with the lid closed, to 180° F.

2. In a shallow baking dish, combine 2 cups water with all ingredients except for the rum and place directly on the grill grate. Smoke for 30 minutes. Grill: 180 °F

3. Remove from the grill and pour into the pitcher of a blender. Process until somewhat frothy.

4. Pour 1.5 ounces of rum each into 4 glasses. Split hot butter mixture evenly between the four glasses.

5. Garnish with a cinnamon stick and freshly grated nutmeg. Enjoy!

Printed in the USA
CPSIA information can be obtained
at www.ICGtesting.com
LVHW081203220624
783646LV00006B/372